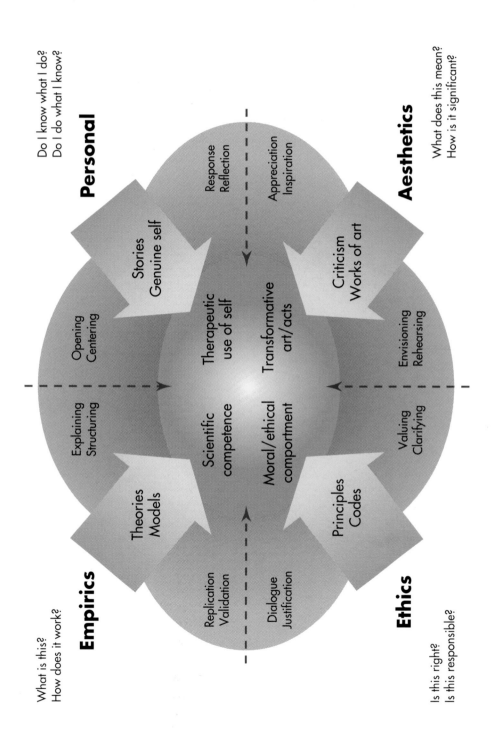

Personal

Do I know what I do?
Do I do what I know?

Aesthetics

What does this mean?
How is it significant?

Empirics

What is this?
How does it work?

Ethics

Is this right?
Is this responsible?

Response
Reflection

Appreciation
Inspiration

Stories
Genuine self

Criticism
Works of art

Opening
Centering

Therapeutic
use of self

Transformative
art/acts

Envisioning
Rehearsing

Explaining
Structuring

Scientific
competence

Moral/ethical
comportment

Valuing
Clarifying

Theories
Models

Principles
Codes

Replication
Validation

Dialogue
Justification

THEORY AND NURSING
INTEGRATED KNOWLEDGE DEVELOPMENT

Peggy L. Chinn, RN, PhD, FAAN

Professor of Nursing
University of Connecticut School of Nursing
Storrs, Connecticut

Maeona K. Kramer, RN, PhD

Professor of Nursing
University of Utah
Salt Lake City, Utah

FIFTH EDITION

with 12 illustrations

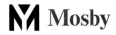 Mosby

St. Louis Baltimore Boston Carlsbad Chicago Minneapolis New York Philadelphia Portland
London Milan Sydney Tokyo Toronto

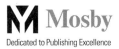

Mosby

Dedicated to Publishing Excellence

Publisher: Sally Schrefer
Editor: Yvonne Alexopoulos
Associate Developmental Editor: Melissa K. Boyle
Project Manager: Deborah L. Vogel
Production Editor: Karen L. Allman
Designer: Bill Drone
Manufacturing Manager: Linda Ierardi
Cover Designer: Pati Pye

FIFTH EDITION

Composition by Graphic World, Inc.
Printing/binding by Maple-Vail Book Mfg Group

Mosby, Inc.
11830 Westline Industrial Drive
St. Louis, Missouri 63146

Library of Congress Cataloging-in-Publication Data
Chinn, Peggy L.
    Theory and nursing : integrated knowledge development / Peggy L. Chinn, Maeona K. Kramer—5th ed.
    p. cm.
    Includes bibliographical references and index.
    ISBN 0-323-00317-6
    1. Nursing—Philosophy.   I. Kramer, Maeona K.   II. Title.
    RT84.5 C487 1998
    610.73′01—dc21
                                             98-31652
                                              CIP

98 99 00 01 02/9 8 7 6 5 4 3 2 1

Reviewers

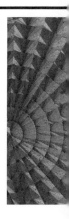

Patricia S. Jones, PhD, RN
Professor
School of Nursing
Loma Linda University
Loma Linda, California

Jeanne Sorrell, PhD, RN
Associate Professor
College of Nursing and Health Science
George Mason University
Fairfax, Virginia

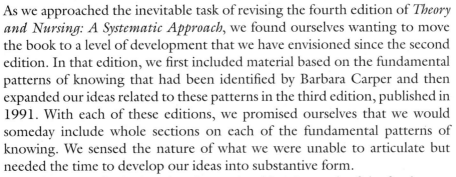

Preface

As we approached the inevitable task of revising the fourth edition of *Theory and Nursing: A Systematic Approach*, we found ourselves wanting to move the book to a level of development that we have envisioned since the second edition. In that edition, we first included material based on the fundamental patterns of knowing that had been identified by Barbara Carper and then expanded our ideas related to these patterns in the third edition, published in 1991. With each of these editions, we promised ourselves that we would someday include whole sections on each of the fundamental patterns of knowing. We sensed the nature of what we were unable to articulate but needed the time to develop our ideas into substantive form.

Realizing our limitations in adequately addressing each of the fundamental patterns of knowing, and also realizing that as yet we had little to draw on within the discipline, in 1990 we each began investigations that could eventually result in substantially new material for a new edition of this book. Peggy conducted what she calls an "aesthetic inquiry" project (Chinn, 1994, 1997), which resulted in new insights related to aesthetic knowing and the art of nursing, as well as new insights related to personal knowing. Maeona began an historical investigation of early nursing literature to identify conceptual meanings for each of the fundamental patterns of knowing.

Although we acknowledge that our prior editions of *Theory and Nursing: A Systematic Approach* were important contributions to the nursing literature, as we approached this revision, we decided, with some trepidation, that it was time to realize our vision of a more complete description of knowledge development in nursing. We had, and still have, some reservations about our readiness to provide adequate descriptions of knowledge development methods for all of the fundamental patterns of knowing, but we harbor a deep commitment to broaden the concepts of knowledge and knowing in nursing. We could no longer claim that nursing depends on patterns of knowing beyond that of empirics and neglect to address these other patterns in some significant manner. Thus a fifth edition of *Theory and Nursing: A Systematic Approach* was not to be. In *Theory and Nursing: Integrated Knowledge Development* we have taken the leap into territory that is not yet fully developed or understood. However, we offer our ideas as a resource for seriously embracing the full extent of knowledge upon which nursing practice is founded and for taking seriously the work that is required to develop this knowledge.

Admittedly, despite our commitment to address more fully each of the fundamental patterns of knowing, our developing ideas remain uneven. Undoubtedly, as an astute reader you will notice that the majority of the chapters are devoted to the empiric pattern of knowing and that each of the other patterns of knowing is addressed in its own relatively brief chapter. Part of our personal work in completing this revision was to develop a level of comfort with our uneven expertise. We resolved this by viewing this book as a "bridge effort" that would extend to the nursing community the ideas we have developed to date, shared in the best form possible.

Naming is a powerful tool. Once something is named, it becomes real. Once real, it can be inspected, scrutinized, critiqued, and understood. Thus naming our ideas seemed an important initial step. It is our expectation that the ideas we have begun to formulate will continue to develop and that the next edition will be more complete. We expect that more complete and better conceptualizations of knowing and knowledge will emerge as the bridge to subsequent editions is crossed. We invite you to share in this ongoing development of ideas and use the ideas we have presented here to stimulate your own ideas and your own work that can contribute to this collective project of conceptualizing nursing knowledge.

Chapter 1 continues to focus on nursing's patterns of knowing. In this chapter we present a new model that overviews the essential interrelationships between knowing and knowledge in nursing for each pattern and as a whole. In this chapter you will encounter new terminology and ideas that build on our prior conceptualizations of the processes for developing nursing knowledge but that now convey links between knowing and doing, knowledge and practice, knowledge and knowing.

Chapter 2 contains the material from the previous edition's Chapter 3. This chapter overviews the historical development of nursing with a particular focus on knowledge development. Although this chapter is similar to that in previous editions, we have added discussion of how each of the patterns of knowing is reflected historically, based on Maeona's scrutiny of the early literature.

Chapters 3, 4, 5, and 6 contain the classic content on theory development from prior editions. Although this edition no longer uses the system for theory development as a major organizing focus, we have retained essential elements of the previous system. Chapter 3 describes the processes of explaining and structuring theory and includes the processes of creating conceptual meaning and structuring and contextualizing theory. The previous edition's Chapters 8 and 9 are now contained in Chapters 5 and 6. Chapter 5 focuses on replicating and validating empiric knowledge through research, and Chapter 6 on replicating and validating empiric knowledge through practice. Chapters 5 and 6 include the previous system activities of generating and testing theoretic relationships and deliberately applying theory. The much beloved chapters from our previous editions that covered the description and critical reflection of theory are merged in Chapter 4 of this edition.

Lest the details of this shifting become a burden, let us summarize. You will find the material formerly located in Chapters 2 and 4 through 9 revised and rearranged around the new model for knowledge development but retained essentially intact in Chapters 3 through 6 of *Theory and Nursing: Integrated Knowledge Development,* with appropriate revisions to reflect our current thinking. These chapters in this edition also contain a small but significant amount of new material that enhances the conception of empiric knowing as a part of the whole of knowing.

Chapters 7, 8, and 9 address knowledge development within the patterns of ethics, personal knowing, and aesthetics, respectively. By giving each of these patterns a chapter, we have detailed, as fully as we could, the ontology and epistemology of each pattern with our new model for knowledge development as a template. You will especially benefit from Peggy's work to describe a method for developing aesthetic knowledge; this chapter is the most developed of these three new chapters. Because of a close link between aesthetic and personal knowing, Peggy's work also led to a number of important insights related to the development of personal knowledge. However, the chapters on personal knowing and ethics are less developed, reflecting the status of our work to date.

Finally, we have included an epilogue. Here we abandon the more formal discourse characteristic of textbooks and share, from our hearts, our commitment to the development of all knowing patterns and our motivations for struggling with the development of the material you find within these pages.

We have provided in this edition an updated glossary, reflecting the ongoing challenge of keeping word definitions current and adding new words that are in our new model. The previous Appendix A, which overviews important broad conceptual models and frameworks in nursing, and Appendix B, which provides examples of midrange theory, have been retained. We retained these unchanged based on reader comments, which indicated they were valuable. Their purpose remains to provide illustrative summaries of some of nursing's theoretical writings.

NOTATIONS ON LANGUAGE

We continue to work on language shifts that reflect our personal values and the values of nursing. We still find, despite an overarching vigilance, words with subtle and blatant meanings that contradict these values. Because these language changes and their inherent value shifts are not easily recognized, we include here notations on the deliberate language changes that first appeared in the third edition.

Our initial aim was to shift the writing style to a clearer, more accessible, and more readable form. From reader comments we believe we have had some success in this area. We have always maintained that language needs to be a vehicle for healing within the profession and should connect those who develop knowledge with those who utilize knowledge. Until we no longer need a language that identifies nurses as academics or practitioners, nurses who work in academia and nurses who work in practice need to communicate better with one another. Consistent with this commitment, we began the editing process with the intent to eliminate words and phrases that depended on or assumed a style typically reserved for the academician. We began by simplifying the sentence structure, eliminating pretentious words when a common word would do, shifting to the active voice as much as possible, and limiting the use of pronouns to instances when an agent is clearly identifiable.

As we worked, we became aware of more flaws in the underlying structure of the language and tried to address them as consistently as possible. We became conscious of value assumptions and connotations that were inherent in the language. Many of the terms that are commonly associated with the practice of scientific methods carry antagonistic, adversarial, objectifying, and militaristic connotations that are contrary to the intents of a human science. Some terms we found to occur with impressive frequency were *competing images, judgments, capture, aim, target, operation, boundaries, argument,* and *debate.* Even when the strict meaning of a word was adequate for the text, we sought to shift the language to words that carry a similar literal meaning but a more human and caring value connotation. For example, instead of the phrase "argue your position," we use "share your ideas."

There were other subtle meanings that we had built into the language and structure of earlier editions of the book, some of which were contradictory to our intent. We did not intend to prescribe "set" or "best" metatheoretical approaches or to convey a strict adherence to linearity. Yet the semantic structure of much of what we presented resulted in an approach that was authoritarian, prescriptive, and linear. In later editions we shifted from a prescriptive, criteria-based approach to theory description and evaluation, to a mode of questioning and considering alternatives. We have continued to refine and enhance this approach. We deleted references to the "first," "second," or "third" "step" in a process and wrote instead of issues or alternatives that could be addressed in the context of process.

Another shift we made in the language is informed by our intent to reframe traditional relationships between people. We have sought to directly engage and empower the reader. We speak directly to the reader as "you," with the intent to encourage your own abilities and ideas rather than impose the authoritative voice of the text.

In this new edition, where we introduce our ideas about personal and aesthetic knowing and knowledge, the problem of language once again surfaced. We have tried to make this content accessible and understandable. Yet we realize that language that effectively expresses some of these more elusive ideas is not readily available. We hope that our struggles to make these ideas accessible will ultimately reflect a language that will be clear and concise, yet rich with meaning.

The language shifts we have made and continue to make have led to profound differences in how we think about the processes for developing knowledge. We invite you to join us in the process of deepening your understanding and awareness of the ways in which language creates and shapes our collective values, knowledge, and, indeed, our reality.

IN THANKS

When we first conceived the essential elements of this book, we had both recently completed our doctoral education and were entering our academic careers. We are both now in our third decade of teaching and continue our personal growth. We owe much of our maturing abilities to the many who have enrolled in our classes and labored with us to push the edges of knowledge and venture into that which is possible but not yet fully real. It is to each of you who have worked with us in classrooms that we owe our greatest debt of gratitude. Without your continual prodding for clearer explanations, your insistence in pushing us beyond our preconceived notions, much of what has emerged in this book would not have been possible. Indeed, in the classroom you became our teachers, and we give to you our deepest appreciation.

Our many academic colleagues, both within the institutions where we have taught and around the world, have contributed to our thinking by being an informed, critical, and thoughtful audience. Our close friends and chosen families have continued to provide the love and support so essential to this type of work—our deepest thanks and gratitude to you.

As much as we feel deeply the ways in which this work depends on our interactions with each of our colleagues, we acknowledge that the content of this book remains our own doing and our own responsibility. We continue to provide for one another the challenges and the grounding that are inherent in cowriting a work of this type. It is our mutual respect and appreciation that sustains this type of relationship over time, and we are grateful for these mutual gifts. We offer this work to you in the hope that it will continue to provide a perspective that deepens your understanding and inspires your own thoughts and actions.

Peggy L. Chinn *Maeona K. Kramer*

Reference List

Chinn PL: Developing a method for aesthetic knowing in nursing. In Chinn PL, Watson J: *An anthology on art and aesthetics in nursing,* New York, 1994, National League for Nursing.

Chinn PL, Maeve K, Bostick C: Aesthetic inquiry and the art of nursing, *Sch Inq Nurs Prac* 11(2):83-96, 1997.

Contents in Brief

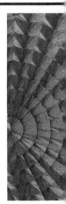

Contents

Chapter 5

Chapter 6

Chapter 1

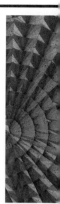

Nursing's Fundamental Patterns of Knowing

It is the general conception of any field of inquiry that ultimately determines the kind of knowledge that field aims to develop as well as the manner in which that knowledge is to be organized, tested and applied. . . . Such an understanding . . . involves critical attention to the question of what it means to know and what kinds of knowledge are held to be of most value in the discipline of nursing.

Barbara A. Carper (1978, p. 13)

Knowing and knowledge are reflections of four patterns: empirics, aesthetics, ethical, and personal. Together they form an essential whole. Praxis—thoughtful reflection and action that occur in synchrony—comes from the whole of knowing and knowledge in nursing practice. This chapter presents a conception of the whole of knowing and knowledge in nursing.

KNOWING AND KNOWLEDGE

In this text, we use the term *knowing* to refer to ways of perceiving and understanding the self and the world. Knowing is an ontologic, dynamic, changing process. We use the term *knowledge* to refer to knowing that is in a form that can be shared or communicated with others. Additionally, knowledge represents what is collectively taken to be a reasonably accurate accounting of the world as it is known by the members of the discipline. Knowledge, then, is a representation of knowing that is collectively judged by standards and criteria shared within the nursing community. The ways in which knowledge and knowing are developed are epistemologic concerns that reveal how we come to know and how we acquire shared knowledge in the discipline.

As nurses practice, they know more than they can communicate symbolically or justify as knowledge. Much of what is known is expressed through actions, movements, or sounds. These are the everyday actions or nondiscursive expressions of knowing that always reflect the whole of knowing. Each of the patterns of knowing has nondiscursive forms of expression that give nursing its distinctive character as a healing practice and that can be recognized as arising from a particular pattern of knowing. At the same time, what is expressed in a nurse's actions always conveys a simultaneous wholeness. Actions also convey a fuller expression of what is known than the formal, discursive expressions of knowledge. Others can observe and comprehend action as a whole, but direct observation is accessible only to those who observe a particular scenario and is therefore limited in serving as a means for communicating what is known to the broader audience of the discipline.

We believe that much of what nurses know has potential to become formally expressed. Although language and other symbols will only partially reflect the whole of knowing, it is important to begin the challenge of formal expression of knowledge in order to communicate what is known within the discipline as a whole. This makes it possible to focus, shape, question, and influence what is collectively accepted as sound, useful, and valued. It is the formal expressions that have potential to become the knowledge of the discipline. Sharing knowledge is important because it creates a disciplinary community, beyond the isolation of individual experience. Once this happens, social purposes form, and knowledge development and shared purposes form a cyclic interrelationship that moves us toward prospective, value-grounded change or praxis.

We have organized this text to focus on processes for development of discursive disciplinary knowledge for nursing praxis, drawing on each of four patterns of knowing within nursing. The methods for developing knowledge are unique to each of the patterns of knowing. The methods that are required for one pattern cannot be used to develop knowledge within another pattern. The scientific methods of empirics, for example, cannot be used to develop personal, ethical, or aesthetic knowledge. This is a challenging ontologic-epistemologic paradox, for the experience of knowing always draws the knower into the whole, where one aspect cannot be comprehended without immediate grasp of the whole of knowing. For example, the methods of science can be described and applied uniquely to the development of empiric knowledge. In the actual experience of scientific inquiry, however, the scientist's personal, ethical, and aesthetic knowing shapes and influences how the inquiry unfolds.

While we discuss the unique features of developing the knowledge of each fundamental pattern, we return again and again to the complementarity of each process and to the aspects of the whole of knowing that influence the unfolding knowledge development process. In the next section we present a conceptualization of the fundamental patterns of knowing that serves as an organizing framework for the entire text. This chapter includes an overview of (1) the essential nature of each pattern in relation to the whole, (2) knowledge development processes within each pattern, and (3) the importance of developing knowledge within all of the fundamental patterns of knowing.

OVERVIEW OF NURSING'S FUNDAMENTAL PATTERNS OF KNOWING

Since Nightingale first established formal education for nurses, nursing has depended on formal knowledge as a basis for practice. The nature of knowledge seen as valuable for nursing changes with time, yet overall the whole of knowledge and knowing that guides and constitutes practice has remained remarkably stable.

Carper (1978) examined early nursing literature and named four fundamental and enduring patterns of knowing that nurses have valued and used in practice. One of the patterns is the familiar and respected pattern of empirics, the science of nursing. In addition, she identified ethics, the component of moral knowledge in nursing; aesthetics, the art of nursing; and personal knowing in nursing.

Other authors have proposed viable additions or adaptations to Carper's conception (Munhall, 1993; Silva, Sorrell, & Sorrell, 1995; White, 1995; Wolfer, 1993). Each of the proposed adaptations to Carper's conception makes a valuable contribution to understanding knowledge and knowing in nursing, and each can be embraced. The patterns that Carper identified remain the fundamental patterns that were reflected in nursing's early literature and have endured as essential aspects of nursing knowledge for more than a century. The fundamental patterns do not exclude other conceptualizations of knowing, and with time certain adaptations to nursing's fundamental knowledge will emerge in new directions.

The fundamental patterns of knowing remain valuable in that they conceptualize a broad scope of knowing that accounts for a holistic practice. We retain our focus on these fundamental patterns in this text because until very recently the development of empiric knowledge has been the prevailing approach to knowledge development, and the other fundamental patterns have not been formally developed within the discipline. In part, neglect of the personal, ethical, and aesthetic patterns of knowing reflects an overvaluing of empirics as the knowledge of the discipline. In addition, methods for developing knowledge within the other patterns, particularly personal and aesthetic knowledge, are only beginning to be systematically described and developed.

In the following sections we describe each of the fundamental patterns and provide an overview of the methods we propose for developing each of the patterns.

Empirics: The Science of Nursing

Empirics is based on the assumption that what is known is accessible through the senses: seeing, touching, hearing, and so forth. Empirics can be traced to Nightingale's precepts concerning the importance of accurate observation and record keeping. The science of nursing emerged during the late 1950s (Carper, 1978). Empirics as a pattern of knowing draws on traditional ideas of science in which reality is viewed as something that can be known by observation and verified by other observers.

Empiric knowing is expressed in practice through the nurse's scientific competence—embodied knowing that makes possible competent action grounded in scientific theory. There is a cognitive component of empiric competence that involves problem solving and logical reasoning, but much of the underlying empiric knowing that informs competent reasoning remains in the background of conscious awareness. It is also accessible to conscious reasoning when attention turns to the reasoning process itself.

Empiric knowledge is formally expressed in the form of empiric theories, statements of fact, or descriptions of empiric events or objects. The development of empiric knowledge has traditionally been accomplished by the methods of science. Usually this has involved testing hypotheses derived from a theory that offers a tentative explanation of empiric phenomena. Although many conceptualizations of empiric knowledge in nursing are linked to this traditional view of science, ideas about what is legitimate for developing the science of nursing have broadened to include activities that are not strictly within the realm of hypothesis testing, such as phenomenologic or ethnographic descriptions or inductive means of generating theory.

Ethics: The Moral Component of Knowledge in Nursing

Ethics in nursing is focused on matters of obligation or what ought to be done. The moral component of knowing in nursing goes beyond knowledge of the norms or ethical codes of nursing, other related disciplines, and society; it involves making moment-to-moment judgments about what ought to be done, what is good and right, and what is responsible. Ethical knowing guides and directs how nurses conduct their practice, what they select as important, where loyalties are placed, and what priorities demand advocacy.

Ethical knowing also involves confronting and resolving conflicting values, norms, interests, or principles. There may be no satisfactory answer to an ethical dilemma or moral distress—only alternatives, some of which are more or less satisfactory. Ethical knowing in nursing requires both an experiential knowledge, from which ethical reasoning arises, and knowledge of the formal principles, ethical codes, and theories of the discipline and society (Carper, 1978). Like empiric knowing, ethical knowing is expressed in nursing actions—what we call moral-ethical comportment. Nursing actions based on ethical knowing can be observed by others, and the underlying ethical principles can be discerned and examined.

The discipline's ethical principles, codes, and theories are set forth in the philosophic ideals on which ethical decisions rest. Ethical knowledge does not describe or prescribe what a decision or action should be; rather, it provides insight about which choices are possible and why, and it provides direction toward choices that are sound, good, responsible, or just.

Ethical theories are like empiric theories in that they describe some dimensions of reality and express relationships between phenomena. However, empiric theory relies on observable reality that can be confirmed by others. Ethical theory cannot be tested in this sense because the relationships of the theory rest on underlying philosophic reasoning that leads to conclusions concerning what is right, good, responsible, or just. The reasoning can include description of experience to substantiate an argument, but the conclusions are value statements that cannot be perceived or confirmed empirically.

Personal Knowing in Nursing

Personal knowing in nursing concerns the inner experience of becoming a whole, aware, genuine self. Personal knowing encompasses knowing one's own self and the self of others. As Carper (1978, p. 18) stated, "One does not know about the self, one strives simply to know the self." It is through knowing one's own self that one is able to know the other. Full awareness of the self, the moment, and the context of interaction makes possible meaningful, shared human experience. Without this component of knowing, the idea of therapeutic use of self in nursing would not be possible (Carper, 1978).

Personal knowing is most fully communicated as an authentic, aware, genuine self. What is perceived by others is the existence of a person, an embodied self. As personal knowing emerges more fully throughout life, the unique or genuine self can be more fully expressed and becomes accessible as a means by which deliberate action and interaction take form. It is possible to describe certain things about the self in personal stories and autobiographies. These descriptions provide sources for deep reflection and a shared understanding of how personal knowledge can be developed and used in a deliberative way. Descriptions about the self are limited in that they never fully reflect personal knowing, and they are retrospective in that they can describe only the self that was. However, publicly expressed descriptions can be a tool for developing self-awareness and self-intimacy and for communicating to others valuable possibilities for developing personal knowing (Hagan, 1990; Nelson, 1994).

In a sense, all knowing is personal; each individual can know only through their personal senses and sensibilities. Empiric theories can be learned, but their meaning for the individual comes from personal reflection and experience with the phenomena of the theory. Aesthetic sensibilities, ethical precepts, and moral beliefs are likewise highly personal in nature. We recognize this broad meaning of personal knowing, but our focus is the aspect of personal knowing that delves into the processes of knowing the self and of developing self-knowing through healing encounters with others.

Aesthetics: The Art of Nursing

Aesthetic knowing in nursing involves deep appreciation of the meaning of a situation, calling forth inner creative resources that transform experience into what is not yet real but possible. Aesthetic knowing makes it possible to move beyond the surface—beyond the limits and circumstances of a particular moment—to sense the meaning of the moment and connect with depths of human experience that are common but unique in each experience (sickness, suffering, recovery, birth, death). Aesthetic knowing in nursing is made visible through the actions, bearing, conduct, attitudes, narrative, and interactions of the nurse in relation to others. It is also expressed in art forms such as poetry, drawings, stories, and music that reflect and communicate symbolic meanings embedded in nursing practice.

Aesthetic knowing is what makes possible knowing what to do with—and how to be in—the moment, instantly, without conscious deliberation. It arises from a direct perception of what is significant in the moment—that is, grasping meaning in the encounter. Perception of meaning in an encounter creates artful nursing action, and the nurse's perception of meaning is reflected in the action taken (Carper, 1978). The meaning is often a shared meaning that is perceived without conscious exchange of words and may not be consciously or cognitively formed. Sometimes meaning is brought to the situation from the nurse's own creative sensibilities, opening possibilities that would not otherwise enter into the encounter. The actions— movements and verbal expressions—of the nurse serve to transform and shape the experience into what would not otherwise exist, creating new possibilities in the encounter. The nurse's actions take on an element of artistry, creating unique, meaningful, deeply moving interactions with others that touch common chords of human experience. We refer to this aspect of nursing practice as the transformative art-act.

Aesthetic knowing is expressed in the moment of experience-action (Benner, 1984; Benner and Wrubel, 1989), in the transformative art-act. Aesthetic knowledge is formally expressed in aesthetic criticism and in works of art that symbolize experience. Aesthetic criticism is the discursive expression of aesthetic knowledge that conveys the artful aspects of the art, the technical skill required to perform the art-act, knowledge that informs the development of the art-act, the historical and cultural significance of specific aspects of nursing as an art, and the potential for the future development of the art.

PROCESSES FOR DEVELOPING NURSING KNOWLEDGE

Nursing's patterns of knowing are interrelated and arise from the whole of experience. Nurses learn a portion of the knowledge of the discipline in their basic education and continue to build on their acquired knowledge as they practice (Benner, 1984). In addition to the knowledge that is acquired through formal and informal education, the experience of practice forms dimensions of knowing. What is known through the experience of practice is reflected in the practice and contributes to the development of formally expressed nursing knowledge. Formally expressed nursing knowledge is developed by using methods of inquiry that are grounded in both practice and formal scholarly methods specifically designed for each pattern.

Figure 1-1 is a representation of how the unique processes and expressions of each pattern contribute to the whole of knowing. In the figure, each of the fundamental patterns is represented in a quadrant. At the periphery of each quadrant are critical questions that each pattern addresses. In the center of each quadrant, a large arrow represents the forms of expression of knowledge within each pattern. The arrow points to the inner

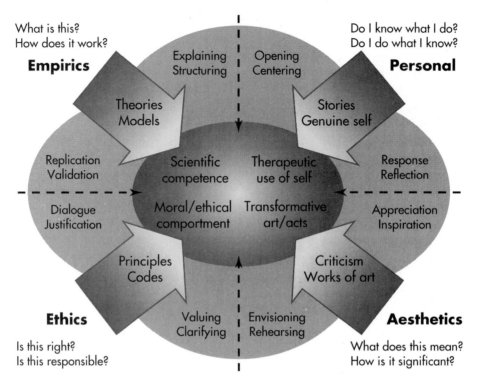

FIGURE 1-1 The processes for developing nursing knowledge.

sphere, showing the practice or action expression of knowing that is associated with the pattern. The inner sphere is shown as a whole, without quadrant boundaries, representing our view that in nursing practice knowing is experienced as a whole and cannot be experienced as discrete patterns. Along the vertical axis, represented by vertical broken arrows, are the processes for developing the formal knowledge expressions. Along the horizontal axis, represented by horizontal broken arrows, are the collective processes used within the discipline for validating or authenticating what is known.

The outer area, where the critical questions appear, and the inner sphere, showing the action expressions of knowing, represent the ontologic dimensions of knowing. The processes shown along the vertical and horizontal arrows represent the epistemologic dimensions of processes for developing and authenticating knowledge.

Another way of conceptualizing these processes is shown in Table 1-1. The dimensions of the critical questions, the creative processes for

TABLE 1-1 Dimensions Associated with Each of the Fundamental Patterns of Knowing

Dimension	Empirics	Ethics	Personal	Aesthetics
Critical questions	What is this? How does it work?	Is this right? Is this responsible?	Do I know what I do? Do I do what I know?	What does this mean? How is it significant?
Creative processes	Explaining, structuring	Valuing, clarifying	Opening, centering	Envisioning, rehearsing
Formal expression of knowledge	Facts, models, theories, descriptions	Principles, codes, ethical theories	Autobiographical stories, the genuine self	Aesthetic criticism, works of art
Authentication processes	Replication, validation	Dialogue, justification	Response, reflection	Appreciation, inspiration
Nondiscursive expression of knowing in practice	Scientific competence	Moral-ethical comportment	Therapeutic use of self	Transformative art/ acts

developing knowledge, the formal expression of knowledge, the processes for authenticating knowledge, and the nondiscursive expressions of knowing in practice are shown for each pattern. Each of the dimensions are unique to each pattern of knowing; you cannot create empiric theory, for example, by using the creative processes of ethics, personal, or aesthetic knowing. However, in the realm of nondiscursive expression of knowing in practice, knowing is experienced as a whole, even though you can discern those aspects of practice that are possible because of each fundamental pattern of knowing.

Critical questions represent the kind of understanding that emerges within the individual patterns. Empirics, the science of nursing, poses the critical questions "What is this?" and "How does it work?" Personal knowing poses the critical questions "Do I know what I do?" and "Do I do what I know?" Ethics poses the critical questions "Is this right?" and "Is this responsible?" Aesthetics poses the critical questions "What does this mean?" and "How is this significant?"

The creative inquiry processes lead toward formal expression of knowledge. Empiric knowledge development uses the reasoning processes of explaining and structuring empirical phenomena. Personal knowledge is developed by opening and centering the self. Development of ethical knowledge uses processes of clarifying and valuing issues of rights and responsibilities in practice. Aesthetic knowledge is developed by envisioning possibilities and rehearsing art-acts that can be called upon to transform experience.

From these processes, formal discursive forms of expression are created that can be presented to members of the discipline. In Figure 1-1, these are shown in the large arrows leading to the center sphere. Empiric inquiry leads to the development of theories, models, and other formal expressions, such as statements of fact and conceptual frameworks. Personal inquiry leads to the creation of autobiographic stories and the lived expression of the nurse's being in nursing care situations. This lived experience of being who we are is what we call the genuine self. Ethical inquiry leads to ethical principles and codes and to other expressions such as theories and precepts that guide ethical conduct in practice. Aesthetic inquiry leads to aesthetic criticism that reveals deep meaning embedded in nursing art-acts and works of art that symbolize nursing experience.

The formal expressions of each pattern, once they are available to the members of the discipline, make possible certain kinds of formal inquiry processes that depend on the community or on the collective efforts of several members of the discipline. These are the processes for authenticating knowledge, represented in Figure 1-1 along the horizontal axis. In the empiric pattern, statements representing empiric reality are translated into inquiry statements that can be replicated in similar but different situations, and the adequacy of the statement can be validated in these similar but different situations. Autobiographic stories and the expression of the genuine self lead to reflection and response from others in the discipline with the intent of discerning the value and adequacy of personal insights. Ethical principles and codes lead to collective dialogue and justification of the soundness of the principles in addressing nursing's ethical and moral dilemmas. Aesthetic criticism and works of art lead to formation of collective appreciation of aesthetic meanings in practice and becomes a source of inspiration for development of the art of nursing.

The innermost sphere in Figure 1-1 represents the nondiscursive forms of expression of knowing that are enacted in the practice of nursing. The nondiscursive expressions represent nursing praxis—the synchrony of thoughtful reflection and action that constitutes nursing as a human caring practice. Praxis assures, through reflections, the continual asking of critical questions associated with each fundamental pattern of knowing, as well as ongoing knowledge development.

All of these processes are interactive and nonlinear, and there is no one starting point. Nurses in practice and nurses who primarily engage in the formal inquiry processes all contribute to the activities that are involved in creating nursing knowledge. Each nurse engages in activities that make possible scientific competence, moral-ethical comportment, therapeutic use of self, and transformative art-acts.

To illustrate how these processes interact, suppose you have an empiric problem concerning what nursing approaches to relieving pain are effective in practice, and why. You might begin by planning a research program to systematically study two different approaches to pain relief. You would identify the theoretical explanations associated with each approach and plan research studies that test selected hypothetical relationships. Whereas the empiric questions are the starting point and remain the focus of your method, your approaches and methods are influenced by aesthetic meanings of experiences of relieving pain and suffering, personal meanings concerning the experience of pain, and ethical values that influence how and when pain relief is given and received.

Personal knowing is frequently the avenue through which awareness of possibilities that are not yet fully understood first emerges. For example, suppose a nurse comes to realize and appreciate the perspective of a family who is receiving care in the clinic. Something has not seemed to fit, has not felt right, and a growing appreciation of the family's perspective gradually brings a new perspective. The nurse shares her awareness with the family, and the relationship shifts to bring the family's perspective to the center. Personal knowing is the starting point to bring a situation to awareness, but as you explore your awareness, your knowledge of empiric theories also is used as a tool, within a frame of ethical and aesthetic sensibilities.

Suppose you want to address an ethical question concerning what is right. You might begin with the focused creative activities of making explicit the personal and group values (valuing) that should guide your actions, clarifying the positions you find in ethical theories and principles that inform the issue, and setting forth how the application of these principles would function with the people with whom you work. These processes would lead you to a dialogue and justification of your ideas based primarily in ethical reasoning. When you begin to share your ideas with your colleagues, the questioning and discussion that result will bring to awareness the personal insights of others engaged in the dialogue, empiric evidence about similar situations, and the range of aesthetic meanings that are possible in this and similar situations.

Aesthetics as a starting point, like personal knowing, often begins with a nurse's own awareness, but the expression often takes an art form that shows what the nurse envisions about the situation. The art can be in the form of the nurse's action in a situation. Suppose a nurse feels a connection to a person's experience of chronic pain. In a moment of caring for the person, the nurse acts from a deeply developed knowing of the meaning of chronic pain in a way that connects with the person's own experience, bringing together empiric, personal, and ethical knowing and creating a possibility that was not previously present.

PATTERNS GONE WILD

When knowledge within any one pattern is not critically examined and integrated with the whole of knowing, distortion instead of understanding is produced. Failure to develop knowledge integrated within all of the patterns of knowing leads to uncritical acceptance, narrow interpretation, and partial utilization of knowledge. We call this "the patterns gone wild." When this occurs, the patterns are used in isolation from one another, and the potential for synthesis of the whole is lost.

Empirics removed from the context of the whole of knowing produces control and manipulation. Ironically, these have been explicit traditional goals of the empiric sciences. When the validity of empiric knowledge is not questioned, one danger is its potential use in contexts where it does not belong. When you recognize how all the patterns contribute to the validity of empirics, you begin to see the unquestioned goals of control and manipulation as a distortion or misuse of empiric knowledge.

Ethics removed from the context of the whole of knowing produces rigid doctrine and insensitivity to the rights of others. This happens when someone simply sets forth personal ideas concerning what is right or good and advocates a position on reasoning derived from personal perspectives. The person may present a justification for a perspective to others but not take seriously the processes of dialogue that the justification invites. In the absence of this integrating process, the person's position remains isolated, with little or no opportunity for empiric, personal, or aesthetic insights to give meaning and social relevance to the ideas.

Personal knowing removed from the context of the whole of knowing produces isolation and self-distortion. When this happens, the self remains isolated, and knowledge of self comes only from what is known internally. Self-distortions can take a wide range of forms, from aggrandizement and overestimation of self to destruction and underestimation of self.

Aesthetics removed from the context of the whole of knowing produces indulgence in self-serving expressions and lack of appreciation for the fullness of meaning in a context. Human actions emerge from and are represented by the tastes and desires of the individual alone, without taking into account the deep cultural meanings inherent in the art-act. Art-acts become self-serving, shallow, arrogant, and empty. Self-serving preferences grow out of a failure to comprehend the deeper cultural, historical, and political significance of the art-act itself. Inauthentic meanings are assigned to another's experience, or a self-serving posture is assumed with respect to another person.

To illustrate "patterns gone wild," imagine an elderly woman admitted to a nursing home. She has lived a life rich in experience and activities and loves to verbally explore her past, making sense of what it means and how it relates to her present life. Having always been physically active, she takes a nightly stroll before going to bed. In the nursing home, she climbs over the bed rails after the lights are out and, with her walker, walks the halls, unsteady but determined, smiling and peering into other rooms. Hearing other residents talking or moaning, she sometimes goes into their rooms and tells them stories or talks with them to ease their troubled nights.

Consider what you might see if any one of the patterns of knowing were isolated from the context of the whole of knowing. Empirics isolated from the other patterns of knowing might require giving a drug that would be effective in bringing sleep to the woman soon after the lights go out, thereby controlling the situation and manipulating her into compliance, regardless of any other concerns. Ethics taken alone might impose the nurse's view of what is right or good for the woman and lead to a rule that would confine the woman to her bed after the lights are out and create a rigid, rule-oriented atmosphere that is insensitive to what the woman and others see as right or good. Personal knowing in isolation would impose the nurse's perspective, with the nurse isolated in the view that the old woman is a nuisance who is interfering with the time needed to complete the charting for the night. Aesthetics alone would impose the nurse's own tastes, preferences, and meanings on the situation. The nurse might restrain the woman in her bed and use a tape recorder to play the nurse's favorite new age music without considering whether the woman can hear the music or whether she finds the music soothing or appealing.

When ethics, aesthetics, personal knowing, and empirics come together as a whole, the purposes of developing knowledge and the actions based on that knowledge become more responsible and humane and create liberating choices. A whole understanding of the woman in the nursing home would take into account the woman's own safety and the needs of other residents; her personal life history and that which gives her pleasure; the ethical dimensions of personal empowerment, moral development, and caring for others; the aesthetic meaning of her actions in the cultural context of aging; and the personal perspective of the nurses who care for her. Many choices remain open in addressing this situation, but all of these considerations together would lead to nursing approaches that would differ from any of the approaches taken from one knowing perspective alone.

WHY DEVELOP NURSING'S PATTERNS OF KNOWING?

As is shown in Figure 1-1 and our discussion of it, the fundamental reason for developing a body of knowledge in nursing is for the purpose of creating expert nursing practice. Nursing's unique perspective and the particular contributions nurses bring to care come from the whole of knowing, a wholeness that has survived despite a cultural and contextual dominance of empiric knowing (Fry, 1992). In a sense the discipline of nursing can be viewed as the empiric pattern of knowing gone wild in that the majority of formal knowledge development efforts have focused on empiric knowledge development methods. Moreover, knowledge has been equated with empiric forms to the exclusion of any other forms of expression.

The idea that knowledge development is separate from the realities of practice can be seen as deriving from the dominance of empirics. Empiric theory is inadequate to represent the complexity of the practice world, and the methods of science traditionally have considered the uncontrolled and unpredictable contingencies in the practice realm unacceptable for the purposes of developing empiric knowledge. The practice implications of empiric theory are often not direct or immediately obvious, and empiric theory often uses a different language from that used in practice.

A shift to a balance in knowledge development to reflect each of the patterns of knowing in nursing holds potential to bring the realm of knowledge development and the realm of practice together. Methods for developing aesthetic, personal, and ethical knowing compel immersion within the realm of practice. Giving attention to these aspects of knowledge development shifts how empirics itself is viewed; empirics becomes part of a larger whole, and its value takes on different meaning in this context. In addition, as greater attention is given to methods other than empirics, many of the traditions and assumptions that underlie empiric methods are challenged, opening the way for creating empiric methods that better accommodate the contingencies of practice.

Formally expressed nursing knowledge provides professional and disciplinary identity, which in turn conveys to others what nursing contributes to the health care process. Professional identity that evolves from distinct disciplinary knowledge provides a basis from which nurses can create certain aspects of their practice. Nursing practice has traditionally been controlled by others, and what nurses do is often invisible. The knowledge that forms nursing practice provides a language for talking about the nature of nursing practice and for demonstrating its effectiveness. Once nursing practice is described, it is made visible. Moving to a conceptualization of knowledge that more fully embraces the whole of practice will serve to impart value to what has been intangible. Also, when nursing's effectiveness can be shown, it can be deliberately shaped or controlled by those who practice it.

On an individual level, nursing knowledge can provide self-identity and esteem as a nurse because you will have a firmer base when your ideas are questioned. As you become familiar with the language and processes of knowledge development, you can begin to think about how assumptions, definitions, and relationships within each of the patterns of knowing can be challenged. The study and understanding of knowledge development will provide a basis on which to take risks, to act deliberately, and to improve practice.

Imagine yourself as a nurse who is using massage to ease chronic pain for a hospitalized person. A physician notices that you are using this method of care. Because this is an unfamiliar approach to the physician, she asks you about it. You explain your reasoning, which is based on nursing knowledge. You can provide research evidence of the effectiveness of massage and information about the positive results that this particular person is experiencing. You can explain the ethical dimensions of providing relief from suffering, the aesthetic components of meaning in the situation, and what you have learned about the therapeutic use of self in giving a massage. Your explanation leads to an informed discussion about various approaches to caring for people with pain and why your approach seems to be effective for this person. As other practitioners learn of your knowledge in this area, they seek your consultation in caring for people with pain. Your knowledge of empiric pain theory and what is effective in caring for people with pain, as well as your ethical, aesthetic, and personal knowledge, provides a valuable resource for developing and improving practice.

Nursing's formally expressed body of knowledge also provides the discipline with a coherence of purpose. Coherence of professional purpose is closely linked to professional identity. Coherence of purpose contributes to a collective identity when nurses agree on the general practice domain. The processes of developing nursing's body of knowledge serve as a means for resolving significant disagreements among practitioners about what is to be accomplished. Varying points of view concerning the general purpose of nursing are reflected in the following questions:

- Should nurses address prevention of illness?
- Should nurses treat human responses to illness?
- Should educational programs be structured around nursing process? Nursing diagnosis? Patterns of knowing? Critical thinking?

- Should nurses view health and illness as opposites?
- Can ill or diseased people also be healthy?

As nurses develop individual and collective responses to these questions, our directions for developing knowledge will be clearer, and in turn our knowledge development efforts will contribute to clarifying responses to questions such as these. Nursing knowledge facilitates coherence by examining such questions as a basis for deliberate choices. When nurses examine and agree about professional purposes and develop knowledge related to those purposes, the public and other practitioners will recognize nursing's expertise in relation to that arena. The fact that nurses are responsible for certain situations will be directly and indirectly communicated to society, and professional identity and coherence of purpose will continue to evolve. By shifting to a balance in the development of all the fundamental knowledge patterns, a sense of purpose can develop that is grounded in the whole of knowing that shapes and directs nursing practice.

CONCLUSION

In this chapter we considered nursing's patterns of knowing and introduced ideas about how the whole of knowing emerges. We have described traits of each pattern: empiric, ethical, aesthetic, and personal knowing. We introduced ideas about how the inquiry processes for each pattern form the knowledge of the discipline. The next chapter provides a description of the history of nursing knowledge development. In the chapters that follow, each of the patterns of knowing and its distinct methods are addressed more fully.

Reference List

Benner P: *From novice to expert: excellence and power in clinical nursing practice,* Menlo Park, Calif, 1984, Addison-Wesley.

Benner P, Wrubel J: *The primacy of caring: stress and coping in health and illness,* Menlo Park, Calif, 1989, Addison-Wesley.

Carper BA: Fundamental patterns of knowing in nursing, *Adv Nurs Sci* 1:13, 1978.

Fry ST: Neglect of philosophical inquiry in nursing: cause and effect. In Kikuchi JF, Simmons H, editors: *Philosophic inquiry in nursing,* Newbury Park, Calif, 1992, Sage.

Hagan KL: *Internal affairs: a journalkeeping workbook for intimacy,* New York, 1990, Harper & Row.

Munhall PL: "Unknowing": toward another pattern of knowing in nursing. *Nurs Outlook* 41:125, 1993.

Nelson GL: *Writing and being: taking back our lives through the power of language,* San Diego, 1994, LuraMedia.

Silva MC, Sorrell JM, Sorrell CD: From Carper's patterns of knowing to ways of being: an ontological philosophical shift in nursing, *Adv Nurs Sci* 18:1, 1995.

White J: Patterns of knowing: review, critique, and update, *Adv Nurs Sci* 17:73, 1995.

Wolfer J: Aspects of reality and ways of knowing in nursing: in search of an integrating paradigm, *Image J Nurs Sch* 25:141, 1993.

Chapter 2

Nursing's Knowledge Development Pathways

Life and nursing are products of all conditions, events and actions of yesterday. Life and nursing tomorrow will relate to today.

Dorothy E. Johnson (1965, p. 38)

The various pathways of nursing's knowledge development form a very large subject. In this chapter we discuss only selected aspects, provide a general outline from our perspective, and in a sense "fly over" the rich history that is available for detailed study. Our purpose is to show evidence of threads of continuity in the development of nursing knowledge that support and give credibility to serious inquiry related to each of nursing's fundamental patterns of knowing.

The earliest conceptions of nursing were grounded in a holistic view of health and healing and recognized all aspects of knowing, which included observation and recording of facts, bringing a sense of virtue to the care of the sick, and appreciating the art of nursing. Nursing then shifted toward primary reliance on empirics and care of the physical body as the primary concerns of the discipline, but threads of philosophic and practical commitment to holistic practices and to other patterns of knowing have persisted. As nursing enters the 21st century, we see serious development of holistic approaches to care and to knowledge and development of methods for all patterns of knowing. This chapter recounts pathways through the emergence of the dominance of empirics, highlighting evidence of many patterns of knowing throughout this period.

Before the advent of "modern nursing" as marked by the Nightingale era, nursing existed in many forms that shared a common core. Shifts in meaning for the word *nursing* and the functions of nurses were largely a product of the social order in which nurses found themselves. The history of nursing is vast and closely tied to the history of medicine. Much of our history has been lost, but based on the available evidence we can speculate on what early nursing must have been like.

Nurses, even if not always so named, have played a clear role in the care of the ill since the beginning of recorded history. Nursing has always been linked with a nurturing role toward the infirmed, ill, and less fortunate—a role usually assigned to the women in society. Long before the advent of Nightingale, there is evidence that "nurses" assisted in the routine care of the sick and in some societies independently provided healing care (Achterberg, 1991). The care provided was influenced by the healing tradition within these early societies. Healers such as shamans, midwives, and other folk healers, who often linked disease to the spirit world, used rituals, ceremonies, and charms to dispel evil and invoke good. Plants and herbal remedies were also employed for healing. Nurses both assisted others and were independent providers of care.

With the rise of empiricism, there was a transition from a view of illness as caused by offending the spirits to a view of disease as the result of natural causes. As the meaning of illness changed, nurses were there to provide nurturing, assistive services. The early religious orders offered a respectable avenue for sisters and monks to provide care to the ill and infirm. Less desirable forms of nursing were also provided by the derelicts of society—often a punishment meted out for civil offenses. Nurses also included women who bore primary responsibility for the care of their ill family members.

NIGHTINGALE'S LEGACY

Although nursing as a nurturing, supportive activity has always existed, it was Nightingale who advocated and promoted the need for a uniformly high standard of nursing care that required both education and a certain personal character. Her actions and writings on the subject of nursing and sanitary reforms earned her recognition as the founder of modern nursing. Thus recognition of nursing as a professional endeavor, distinct from medicine, began with Nightingale.

Nightingale spoke with firm conviction about the nature of nursing as a profession distinct from medicine that could provide an avenue for women to make a meaningful contribution to society (Nightingale, 1969, p. 3). In the mid-1800s, women cared for the English sick as daughters, wives, mothers, or maids. These socially prescribed roles influenced Nightingale's conviction that nursing should be a profession for women, but this cultural tradition was secondary to her philosophy. Her primary concern was the more pervasive plight of Victorian women. Women in her era were either poverty-stricken and forced to work at menial labor for long hours, or they were, as was the case with Nightingale, idle ornaments in the households of wealthy husbands or fathers. In either case, there was no avenue in which women could use their "intellect, passion, and moral activity" to benefit society (Nightingale, 1979).

Nightingale spent the first decade of her adult life tormented by a desire to use her productive capacities in a way that would benefit society. She eventually defied the wishes of her family and broke free of the oppressive social prescriptions for her life. She obtained formal training as a nurse with the religious sisters at Kaiserswerth and subsequently agreed to serve in the Crimean War (Nightingale, 1979; Tooley, 1905; Woodham-Smith, 1983). After her service in the war, Nightingale wrote *Notes on Nursing,* in which she set forth the basic premises on which nursing practice was to be based and articulated the proper functions of nursing. Though written for the lay nurses of the time, *Notes* contains timeless wisdom appropriate for today's professional nurses. In her view, nursing required making astute observations of the sick and their environment, recording observations, and developing knowledge about the factors that promote the reparative process (Nightingale, 1969). Nightingale's framework for nursing emphasized the utility of empiric knowledge, and she is recognized for using the statistics she gathered in a way that would further the cause of health care in England and throughout the world.

Firmly committed to the idea that nursing's responsibilities were distinct from those of medicine, Nightingale maintained that the knowledge developed and used by nursing must be distinct from medical knowledge. Medicine, wrote Nightingale, focused on surgical and pharmacologic "cures," a tradition that relied heavily on empiric science. Nursing, however, was broader. Nursing was to be designed to assist nature in healing the patient. This was accomplished by managing the internal and external environment in an assistive way—in a way that was consistent with nature's laws.

In addition to her concept of nursing as assisting the healing of individual patients, she addressed the context of nursing. Nightingale insisted that women who were trained nurses must control and staff early nursing schools and must manage and control nursing practice in homes and hospitals to create a context supportive of nursing's art. Nightingale's influence on nursing education was felt within schools of nursing in England and the United States. The first Nightingale schools were autonomous in their administration, and nurses held decision-making authority over nursing practice in institutions where students learned.

Instruction in these schools emphasized the powers of observation, the necessity of recording observations, and the potential for organizing nursing knowledge gained through observation and recording. Students also learned proper techniques of nursing. Nightingale's strong beliefs about the values that should be cultivated in nursing were reflected in the educational programs of early schools (Barnard & Neal, 1977; Dennis & Prescott, 1985). Nightingale regarded nursing as a calling and vehemently opposed registration as a way to ensure the quality of practitioners. She argued that testing and subsequent registration might ensure a minimal knowledge base but would not guarantee the quality of moral disposition within the individual nurse. Thus Nightingale both understood and advocated that nursing was much more than knowledge of facts and techniques. These were important, but nursing also required a certain ethical and moral disposition view, a certain type of person, and an ability to act artfully. Good nursing also required a realistic view of the sociopolitical context to create a proper setting for nursing.

FROM NIGHTINGALE TO SCIENCE

After the Nightingale era, many forces in society emerged in opposition to her model for schools of nursing. In the United States, the medical care system developed as a capitalist, for-profit business. This system provided the context for rapid technologic development and a complex industrial system to support medical interventions. Early in the 1900s, as the Nightingale era was ending, medical care was taking shape as a science. The sociopolitical view of women during this era influenced nursing's evolution. With industrialization, the concentration of the populace within urban areas, and the push to settle the expanding Western frontier, the number of hospitals increased dramatically.

Physicians and hospital administrators saw women as a source of inexpensive or free nursing labor who could further their economic goals. Many women entered nursing and provided student labor for hospitals in exchange for receiving the apprenticeship training to become nurses. These were working-class women with limited opportunities for education and meaningful work. Once trained for hospital nursing, they found themselves without employment as bountiful supplies of new recruits entered training and filled the staffing positions they once occupied. Thus, nurses were exploited both as students and as experienced workers. They were treated as submissive, obedient, and humble women who were "trained" in correct procedures and techniques and ideally fulfilled their responsibilities to physicians without question. Nurses' positive desire to help people in need, coupled with their relative lack of educational preparation and social or political power, led to an extended period in history when nursing was practiced primarily under the control and direction of medicine (Lovell, 1980).

Despite strong leaders who followed the Nightingale tradition and viewed nursing knowledge as unique, nursing's knowledge has not always been regarded as distinct from medicine. During the early 1900s, when most of the Nightingale-modeled schools in the United States were brought under the control of hospitals, nursing education and practice were transferred from the profession to the control of hospital administrators and physicians (Ashley, 1976). Strong efforts to move nursing to institutions of higher learning were not enough. Consistent with the social history of women, nursing was viewed and treated increasingly as a role supporting and supplementing medicine and certainly not one that required a unique knowledge base (Hughes, 1980; Lovell, 1980). Although training was acceptable, true education for women and nurses was discouraged, discouraging, and limited. Indeed, education would be counterproductive for women who, as nurses, were expected to follow orders and serve the needs and interests of physicians in providing care (Melosh, 1982; Reverby, 1987).

Economic independence for women was not possible until the mid-1900s. Even a woman who earned an income was not able to have a bank account, own property, or conduct financial transactions in her own name. Normal schools were established for the training of teachers, and nursing schools were available for training nurses, but to obtain long-term security, women were required to conform to the role of wife or daughter.

Throughout the early part of the twentieth century, nursing practice was based on rules, principles, and traditions that were passed along through limited apprenticeship forms of education. Nursing practice also included an ever increasing array of delegated medical tasks that were acquired as medical knowledge expanded—tasks performed by nurses as extensions of physicians. Higher education for nurses was not available; thus much of what evolved as nursing knowledge was wisdom that came from years of experience.

Tradition as a basis for nursing practice was perpetuated by the nature of apprenticeship education in nursing (Ashley, 1976). Student nurses were presumed to learn at random through long hours of experience, with limited exposure to lectures or books, and to accept without question the prescriptions of practical techniques. The novice nurse acquired knowledge of what was right and wrong in practice by observing more experienced practitioners and by memorizing facts about the performance of nursing tasks. Nurse recruits also learned what sort of "person" a nurse should be through the imposition of rigid rules that regulated most aspects of behavior, including sleeping, eating, socializing, and dress, both inside and outside the hospital walls. Rules were strictly enforced with severe penalties for those who strayed outside the rule's boundary. Thus nursing was viewed primarily as a nurturing and technical art requiring apprenticeship learning and innate personality traits congruent with the art (Ashley, 1976; Hughes, 1980).

Despite social impediments to the development of nursing knowledge, nursing philosophy and ideology remained committed to the idea that nursing requires a knowledge base for practice distinct from medicine (Abdellah, 1969; Hall, 1964; Henderson, 1964, 1966; Rogers, 1970). This commitment grew from the consistent recognition that, although the goals of nursing and medicine were related, the central goals and functions of nursing required a broader knowledge not provided by medicine or by any other single discipline outside of nursing.

Although social circumstances limited nursing education, early nursing leaders sustained ideals that reflected Nightingale's model of education and practice. Because most nursing service was provided as free labor by students in hospitals, those who graduated and found themselves unemployed secured jobs as independent practitioners who were engaged by families to assist in the care of the sick in homes and in hospitals. Many nurse leaders were active in confronting a wide range of community-based social and health issues of the time, including temperance, freedom for slaves, suffrage for blacks and women, and control of venereal disease. These roles required a view of nursing that was undergirded by a broad view of nursing knowledge and a desire to change the future. These were women for whom technical training did not "take"; despite that training, they saw nursing broadly.

As nurses developed broad, community-based practices, their writings reflected the multiple patterns of knowing in which their practices were grounded. There is substantial evidence that graduate nurses in the early part of the twentieth century had ethical and moral commitments that contributed substantively to improving health conditions in hospitals, homes, and communities. Not only did they develop health knowledge as they practiced, but they were politically committed to finding ways to distribute this knowledge to people who needed it (Wheeler, 1985).

Consistently throughout the early twentieth century, nursing leaders in the United States worked together nationally and internationally in strong connecting networks to call for a social and political ethic that would restore the control of nursing practice to nurses. Margaret Sanger, Lillian Wald, and Lavinia Dock are among those nurses who led this effort. These nurses were challenged by the specific needs of society and independently set about to develop their practice on the basis of what they saw in health care. They observed the circumstances of people in their communities, identified a health-related need, and organized nurses to meet the needs. Integrating ethical commitment with scientific knowledge, they recorded observations and the conclusions they drew from these observations.

Sanger, for example, developed knowledge about reproduction and birth control. Evidencing a moral commitment to women, she fought against great odds to distribute birth control information to women who were desperate to obtain it and established a foundation for family planning programs that remains viable today (Sanger, 1971). Wald became concerned about child care and family health in the context of extremely poor conditions of sanitation in the crowded immigrant tenements of New York City. She established the Henry Street Settlement in New York City, from which she developed concepts of community health nursing and social welfare programs. She developed stations from which safe milk was distributed to families with young children and centers for educating mothers in the care of their families (Silverstein, 1985; Wald, 1971). Dock was an ardent suffragist and pacifist who worked for much of her professional life with Wald at the Henry Street Settlement. She campaigned actively for changes in labor laws that would benefit women and children. Twenty years of her life were devoted to gaining enfranchisement for women in the United States; she reasoned that if women could vote, the oppressive laws that affected them would be changed (Christy, 1969).

Lydia Hall is a more recent example of a nurse who constructed specific philosophic ideas about how nursing should be practiced and implemented this philosophy in practice. Hall established Loeb Center at Montefiore Hospital in New York City, a nursing center where nursing maintains control over the care provided and where people and their families have primary decision-making power over the kind of care that they receive (Hall, 1963). For Hall nursing could not be practiced within the acute care institution but required a different kind of environment to flourish. She wrote that "there is no shortage of nurses, there is a shortage of nursing" (Hall, 1966, p. 49). In her views of nursing Hall explicitly addressed the significance of the person of both the nurse and the patient. For Hall it is finally in a person-to-person dialogue that growth toward health occurs.

PATTERNS OF KNOWING IN THE EARLY LITERATURE

Like contemporary scholars, early nursing leaders developed and used multiple ways of knowing to ground improvements in health care and nursing practice. They were women of strong personal character who lived their ethical convictions that nurses can and should control nursing practice. Their ethical and moral ideals of nursing practice required making detailed observations, recording these observations, and organizing the knowledge that came from their observations. They orchestrated complex practice changes that required a sense of how to maneuver through, interpret, and balance the context in which they found themselves. Thus art was central to their practice. The early literature in nursing is rich with detail about how nursing practice embodies, reflects, and requires multiple ways of knowing. The following sections provide some examples of how early writings address each pattern of knowing.

Empirics

Prior to the era of "science" in the mid-1950s, there was clear recognition of scientific knowledge as a source of power. A physician who addressed the annual meeting of the Michigan Nurses Association acknowledged that scientific knowledge had increased and asked nurses to acknowledge its power and value for producing knowledge. In this particular article the physician cautioned against quackery and portrayed science as a source of legitimate criteria for selection of information provided to patients (Warnshius, 1926). Despite the value for science, the importance of a central focus on the welfare of the client was emphasized.

Empirics was frequently represented as knowledge of underlying principles and techniques associated with nursing. According to Margaret Conrad (1947), a baccalaureate-prepared professor of nursing, this required an understanding of the laws of nature, the principles of physics, chemistry, physiology, and psychology. In other early articles the procedural and technical aspects of nursing were emphasized, including bed making, food tray handling and feeding, carrying out personal hygienic measures such as bed baths and oral hygiene, and managing delegated medical procedures such as drains, catheterizations, enemas, alcohol baths, vital signs, and medication administration (Brigh, 1944; Mountin, 1943). Muriel Burgess (1941), a nursing student, outlined the "facts of care," which included diagnosis; social factors such as heredity, environment, and education; and medical factors such as past history of family and history of present illness, symptom onset, physical examination, and laboratory and x-ray findings. She further noted that the plan should include the progress of the patient and use graphs whenever possible. Treatments prescribed and the continuing plan for care were also important. Genevieve and Roy Bixler (1945), two doctorally prepared educators, addressed the development of empirics and wrote that "the elements of science should be defined and organized, gathered from every science contributing to nursing and arranged in the most convenient order for thought" (p. 730). Bixler and Bixler stated that scientific compartmentalizations were artificial, arbitrary, and to be avoided by nursing science. Nursing science existed apart from practice, but its use in the service of professional practice represented a "new synthesis." Science, they asserted needs to be integrated as an art.

Formal observation was also established as a valued technique and a skill critical for the development of nursing empirics. A 1947 editorial in the *American Journal of Nursing* admonished nurses to develop keen observation skills because "the lack of descriptions or records of nursing care based on actual experience is appalling" (p. 655). Written observations could form the basis for a complete patient study to provide an interpretive picture of present-day nursing ("Changes," 1947). In a speech at a student nurse convention, Blanche Pfefferkorn (1933), who was identified only as a registered nurse, stated that empiric knowledge came from questionnaires, detached observation, and field studies. According to Pfefferkorn, a scientific attitude was important. Scientific knowledge included "facts that were organized into a form or structure that were not dynamic and reports of field studies." Regardless of source, scientific knowledge served as a skeleton and answered questions about what. Good science represented the what well. Pfefferkorn noted the nurse needed to know how, not just what, and stated that field studies could "enliven fact gathering by providing knowledge of how." Agnes Meade (1936), a nurse who wrote an article titled "Training the Senses in Clinical Observation," cautioned about a pitfall of scientific bias: "A distinguishing feature of scientific observation is that the observer knows what is being sought, and to a certain extent what is likely to be found" (p. 540).

In summary, in the early literature the nature and importance of science for nursing were clearly reflected. Information was provided about how empirics is created and displayed. Although scientific-empirical knowledge could come from disciplines outside nursing, there was recognition of the unique nature of nursing science. Principles, facts gleaned from observation, and procedural guides to action were important forms of empirics that were necessary for completing routine hygienic care of patients, as well as delegated medical tasks. Despite the recognition of the value of empirics, the caution that science alone was an inadequate practice guide appears frequently. A physician addressing a graduating class of diploma nurses told them that "the profession of nursing is an art depending upon science. . . . In nursing the art must always predominate though underlying science is important" (Worcester, 1902).

Ethics

Prior to the 1950s ethics was primarily represented as virtues possessed by the nurse. Nurses were expected to be moral individuals, who, it follows, do the right thing. Virtue and responsibility were paramount for nurses. Duty and responsibility to patient included protection, truth telling, and imparting specialized knowledge (Conrad, 1947; De Witt, 1901; Warnshius, 1926). An editorial in the *American Journal of Nursing* noted that "the doctor is responsible for the general conduct of the case, but the nurse is responsible for the honest performance of her own duties" (De Witt, 1901, p. 15). This editorial further noted that "born qualities added to training" was critical for ethical conduct (De Witt, 1901). Duty was often expressed in religious admonitions to love, to live right, and to have faith. Duty was seen as sacred obligation as illustrated by a lay author who wrote "a good nurse will die before admitting she is even tired [for] loyal service is one of the articles of the profession's religion" (Drake, 1934, pp. 137-138). Moral fitness for nursing was important, and moral examinations were recommended. Agnes Riddles (1928), a nurse, stated that "women [read *nurses*] should hold their position only after a moral examination as well as a technical one" (p. 29). Riddles listed a variety of moral infractions attributable to nurses of the time, including lack of consideration for the patient, neglect of aseptic precautions, disrespect for human life, and lack of proper experience in assembling needed nursing materials.

Charlotte Aikins (1915), presumably a nurse educator, outlined an entire curriculum for teaching ethics in *Trained Nurse and Hospital Review.* The curriculum included knowledge of "the customs and laws of the hospital world which she (student) must be admonished to accept meekly" (p. 136) and "personal virtues of importance such as reticence, tact, and discretion in order that she may do no harm" (p. 136). "Health, carriage, voice, manner, habits and general deportment" (p. 136) were also important. During the junior year ethics would cover "handling of supplies and appliances, avoiding accidents, use of good surgical technique, wise use of recreation and holidays, and the necessity of a good conscience" (p. 137). Another early nurse mentioned the need to keep preconceptions and prejudices to a minimum as a part of ethical conduct (Oettinger, 1939).

Paul Johnson (1928), in an address to a statewide gathering of nurses, asked: "What should ethics teach?" He differentiated ethics and morality. Ethics, according to Johnson, is the "science of right conduct" (p. 1085). Ethics investigates "boldly" what this is by "questioning moral tradition, examining moral facts, and searching out moral values" (p. 1085). Ethics requires "careful investigation, open-minded judgment, the practice of reasonableness and intelligent doubting" (p. 1085). Ethical sensitivity, rather than the rules approach of "laying down exact rules for conduct" (p. 1084), was important to cultivate. Such an attitude questions the establishment of rules as the basis for a biomedical ethics and validates a relational perspective for ethical conduct. Johnson's early article also challenges a virtue ethics by differentiating ethics and morality and calling ethics the "science" of right conduct.

Early authors imparted a variety of goals for ethical knowledge and knowing, including protection of patients' privacy and rights, advocacy, and minimization of patients' discomfort and inconvenience. Broader goals were also mentioned, such as increasing tolerance and respect by respecting the individual worth and autonomy and dignity of individuals, assisting in the development of the individual, strengthening society and self, developing economic security, and promoting peace.

In summary, the early periodical literature reflects a view of ethical behavior and comportment as following from individual virtues. Such virtues were evidenced by religious living, self-sacrifice, and a nearly blind duty to others' rules and prescriptions. However, the seeds of relational ethics are found in the questions raised concerning the cost to the individual and the profession of blind adherence to rules and prescriptions. Although most of what is termed *ethical* comes from religious traditions and authoritative trust in others, writers also discussed questioning traditions and making responsible judgments, studying what we doubt, and analyzing and criticizing basic precepts.

Personal

The importance of the person of the nurse is evident in the ethical pattern in that the prevailing ethics of the time called for a virtuous person. However, qualities of person beyond virtue are also found in the early literature. Margaret Conrad (1947), writing about the nature of expert nursing care, recognized the necessity for a well-balanced, integrated personality to contribute to the care of others. Allen Gregg (1940), a physician, in an address to three national nurse meetings, asked nurses to "seek honestly and earnestly to find what really matters to us and what beliefs and convictions we hold" (p. 738). Gregg also redefined *virtue* as "the inner life as well as the outer in consistency of behavior with one's own thoughts and feelings" (p. 740) and further stated that "motives and conduct must harmonize" (p. 740). Motives must be sound, or there is no virtue in the great sense, no independence and no self-confidence (p. 741). The fundamental importance of personal knowledge is acknowledged in that "only when a person is something to herself can she become anything to anybody else" (p. 741). Gregg's article, written in the postwar period and clearly pacifist in tone, recognized that science cannot provide personal knowledge, for "the social wisdom of man does not derive from chemistry and physics and mechanical skill. Decency does not visit our common dwelling place without invitation" (p. 739). Genevieve Noble (1940), writing as a student in "The Spirit of Nursing," emphasized the need for an inherent inner self-discipline rather than an imposed discipline for adequate nursing care. Katherine Oettinger (1939) gave equal importance to personal knowing and empirics by stating that "the personality of the nurse is quite as important as the distinctive facts she learns" (p. 1224).

Important personal characteristics included acceptance of self grounded in self-knowledge and confidence. Personal integrity and honesty as well as enthusiasm, versatility, courageousness, imaginativeness, stability, and emotional diversity were important features of personal knowledge. Such knowledge is created by engagement with life, finding out what really matters, and reflecting on it. Nursing practice requires a depth of personal knowing that acknowledges the validity of feelings, openness to freely discussing feelings, and examining reciprocal emotions in dialogue and relation. A nurse of high personal character evidences an inner and outer harmony and commands respect of self and others. As Oettinger (1939) put it, such a nurse is "free from conscript minds giving conscript thoughts" and is "free to change the status quo" (p. 1244).

Aesthetics

A sense that nursing has an artistic component is clearly evident in early periodical literature. L. F. Simpson (1914), another physician speaking to nurses, stated that "real nursing is an art; and a real nurse is an artist" (p. 133). Conrad (1947) stated that the art of nursing included such things as "knowing what the patient wants before she is asked" (p. 162). It arises from "combining instinct, knowledge and experience" (p. 162). According to Conrad, art depends on imagination and resourcefulness and requires "true perspective" (pp. 162-163). Furthermore, art requires practice, and some nurses "never acquire it" (Simpson, 1914, p. 135). Experience was seen as important to develop aesthetic knowing. As Austin Drake (1934), a layperson, put it: "Circumstances alter cases . . . the nurse adapts her roles at will according to her patient's physical state and particular mode . . . if he is able and desires . . . she talks, otherwise she is silent, intent upon her duties . . . the severity of the illness does not determine this" (pp. 136-137).

Art in the more traditional sense was recognized as important to the art-act of nursing. In 1923 Lois Mossman (1923), an assistant professor of education, acknowledged that "science cannot explain what happens when we respond to beauty of form or motion but the response is pleasurable and influences what we are doing" (p. 318). Mossman asks novice nurses to "experience beauty, to see it in the commonplace, to learn of books, poems, pictures, and music that interpret beauty and draw from them to fit the needs of those we serve" (p. 319). According to Mossman, "Life is rhythmical and lights must be set off by the shadows" (p. 319). Edward Garesche (1927), a Roman Catholic priest, eloquently expressed the elusiveness of assessing our art and the importance of distinguishing it from empirics. He stated: "The service of the learned professions does not bear measuring while it is being rendered" (p. 901).

In summary, the early literature represents aesthetics as a combination of knowledge, experience, intuition, and understanding. Aesthetic knowing was creative and intuitive and consisted of exquisite judgments without conscious awareness but sensed intuitively by unexplained insight and hunches. Aesthetic knowledge was gained through appreciation of the arts and by subjective sensitivity to individual differences. Aesthetic knowing was also gained by personal imitation of those who possess the art. Aesthetic knowing required speculation, imagining, and the superimposition of impressions on facts. The practitioner who had a sincere intentionality and the ability to carry out sophisticated assessment could act artfully. It was through the interpretation of interaction that each succeeding interaction became more meaningful.

THE EMERGENCE OF NURSING AS A SCIENCE

The shift toward a concept of nursing knowledge as predominantly scientific began in the 1950s and took a strong hold in the 1960s. This shift toward knowledge as science produced significant changes in our view of what is important in nursing. Gradually, nursing shifted from a perspective that emphasized technical competence, duty, and womanly virtue to a perspective that focused more on effective nursing practice (Hardy, 1978). The shift toward science, in many ways, was a welcome change from a focus on nursing as the technically competent performance of delegated medical tasks, blind duty, and womanly virtue. The emphasis on science as knowledge was an important step forward. However, this move was at the sacrifice of the development of ethics of individual and collective practice, the development of nurse character, and the artistic and aesthetic dimensions of practice. These other patterns of knowing, so necessary for practice and so evident in nursing's work throughout the ages, were largely neglected until the early 1990s.

The shift toward science as the basis for developing nursing knowledge was influenced by the involvement of nursing in the two world wars during the 1900s. The wars created social circumstances that brought about substantial shifts in roles for women and nurses. During wars, with many men away from their homes, women were freed from constraints and learned to manage their responsibilities in accord with their own priorities and preferences. Many women entered the skilled or unskilled labor force during the years when men were away in battle. Women who were nurses were needed to support the war effort by providing care for the sick and wounded. War-related programs were instituted by the U.S. government to make nursing preparation available to women who agreed to serve in the war (Kalisch and Kalisch, 1978; Kelly and Joel, 1996).

Partly because of the greater demand for technically skilled nurses to serve the war effort, by the decade of World War II women had begun to enter institutions of higher learning in greater numbers. The early nursing leaders' vision of nursing education within colleges and universities began to be realized. After the end of World War II, many educational programs were established within institutions of higher learning, and graduate programs for nurses began to appear. Academic institutions required faculty to hold advanced degrees and encouraged them to meet the standards of higher education with regard to service to community, teaching, and research. Research standards followed the criteria of scientific-empiric work, which limited the nature of credible scholarship among academic nurses. Nurse-scientist programs were established to enable nurses to earn doctoral degrees in other disciplines with the idea that research skill could then be transplanted into nursing. Once nurses gained skills in the methods of science, nursing theories and other types of theoretic writings began to emerge. These conceptualizations of nursing followed the tradition of the disciplines in which doctorally prepared nurses were educated. Yet, these theories of nursing did not follow the rules of traditional scientific theory.

In 1950 *Nursing Research,* the first nursing research journal, was established. Books on research methodologies, and explicit conceptual frameworks, often called "theories of nursing," began to appear. Early research reports were less sophisticated in method than those of today, but these writings changed and began to reflect qualities of serious empiric scholarship and investigative skill. Various schools of thought that emerged about the nature of nursing practice and nursing's knowledge base provided a fresh flow of ideas that could be examined by members of the profession. These writings provided a stimulus for early efforts in developing theory and eventually to broader knowledge-development efforts.

By the 1960s doctoral programs in nursing were being established. By the end of the 1970s the number of doctorally prepared nurses in the United States had grown to nearly 2000. Approximately 20 doctoral programs in nursing had been established, and masters programs were maturing in academic stature and quality. Masters programs were focused on preparing advanced practitioners in nursing rather than on preparing educators and administrators. With the development of advanced educational programs, nurses began to formally consider the processes and ends for development of nursing knowledge. Nurse scholars began to debate ideas, points of view, and methods in the light of nursing's traditions (Hardy, 1978; Leininger, 1976). These debates are reflected in the literature of the late 1960s and early 1970s (Dickoff and James, 1971; Dickoff, James, and Wiedenbach, 1968; Ellis, 1971; Folta, 1971; Walker 1971, Wooldridge, 1971). Fundamental differences in viewpoints about nursing science provided nurse scholars the opportunity to learn, sharpen critical-thinking skills, and acquire knowledge about the processes and limitations of science.

As an overt and deliberative focus on knowledge development began to take shape in nursing, a prevailing view that emerged was that of nursing as a service that required a strong base in science. Debates reflected various views of science and metatheory (theory about knowledge and theory development) and the preferred methods for producing sound nursing knowledge. Despite the lively debates and substantive issues focused on scientific knowledge, the idea that nursing requires development of a broad knowledge base that includes all patterns of knowing has never been lost. Even when this broad view was not explicitly mentioned in the debates (as was common during the 1970s), the broad conceptualizations labeled *theories* implicitly required multiple ways of knowing. The persistent dominance of science can be attributed in part to academic nurses' need to gain legitimacy in their university communities and to nurses' need to achieve political and personal legitimacy within medicine and society in general. Regardless of societal context, the wholistic focus of nursing has endured.

Throughout the second half of the 20th century, three major trends contributed to evolving directions in developing nursing knowledge. These trends, as would be expected, centered on the scientific-empiric pattern. However, there are threads of continuity that reflect ethics, aesthetics, and personal knowing, as we show in the sections that follow. The three trends are (1) application of theories borrowed from other disciplines, (2) development of philosophies and theories defining nursing, and (3) the development of midrange theory linked to practice.

The Application of Theories Borrowed from Other Disciplines

As the educational preparation of nurses expanded, theories developed in other disciplines were recognized as important for nursing. Problems in nursing practice for which there had seemed no ready solution began to be viewed as resolvable if theories from other disciplines were applied. For example, nurses recognized that young children needed the continuing love and support of their parents and families during hospitalization. The strict rules of hospitals that severely restricted visitation interrupted these primary family ties. As psychologic theories of attachment and separation developed, nurses found an explanation for the problems experienced by hospitalized children and were able to change visitation practices to provide sustained contact between parents and children.

Although theories from other disciplines have been useful, nurses have also exercised caution in arbitrarily applying these theories. In some instances, the theories of other disciplines do not take into consideration significant factors that influence a nursing situation. For example, some theories of learning applicable to classroom learning do not adequately reflect the process of learning when an individual is faced with illness. Nor do they deal with the ethical issues a nurse might face in disclosing sensitive information to a patient. Although borrowed theories may be useful, their usefulness cannot be assumed until they are examined from the perspective of nursing in nursing situations (Whall, 1980).

Development of Philosophies and Theories Defining Nursing

As nurses began to reconsider the nature of nursing and the purposes for which nursing exists in light of science, they began to question many ideas that were taken for granted in nursing and the traditional basis on which nursing was practiced. They wrote and published idealized views about nursing and the type of knowledge, skills, and background needed for practice. As an ideal view of nursing, these models and philosophies did not arise from practice per se but did reflect a reasonably attainable vision of what nursing could be. Writings of the 1960s and 1970s made significant contributions to the development of theoretic thinking in nursing. Many have been used as a basis for curricula and as guides for practice and research.

Many early nursing conceptual models and philosophies include a description of the nursing process. This process, which is similar to both scientific methods of problem-solving and research processes, is a framework for viewing nursing as a deliberate, reflective, critical, and self-correcting system. The nursing process replaced the rule- and principle-oriented approaches that were grounded in a medical model in which the nurse functions as a physician's assistant. The nursing process relied heavily on what could be assessed through observation. Prior to a focus on the nursing process, unexamined rules and principles were used to guide the nurse in routine hygienic care, performance of treatment procedures, and administration of medications to treat disease. Because a rule-oriented approach did not encourage reflective problem solving, the shift to the nursing process as a way to approach care encouraged nurses to cultivate basic inquiry skills. Nursing diagnosis, which evolved from the nursing process and began to move nursing away from theoretic dependence on a medical model, was one means for organizing the domain of nursing practice. The early literature concerning nursing diagnosis included both practical and theoretic ideas about developing a taxonomy of nursing diagnoses and testing their validity.

Conceptual models for nursing education and practice proliferated in the 1960s and 1970s. There was considerable debate about whether the writings of such leaders as Callista Roy, Betty Neuman, Imogene King, and Dorothea Orem were termed *models, theories,* or *philosophies,* reflecting an underlying acknowledgment that science alone was an inadequate metatheory for practice. Regardless of labels, nursing practice consistent with these (and other) models was taught in educational institutions, integrated into practice, and undergirding research. The use of nursing models cultivated a tacit recognition of the significance of the aesthetic, ethical, and personal components of nursing knowledge. As nurses began to integrate these ideas into practice settings, the actual and potential relationships between nursing models and nursing practice became clearer. Practicing nurses found a new sense of purpose and direction consistent with the basic values of nursing and a sense of the increasing effectiveness achieved through systematic and thoughtful forms of nursing practice. Transferring these ideals of practice into the health care setting also served to illuminate the difficulties of finding nursing opportunities in the increasingly competitive health care system.

Another early formal movement was defining the discipline by using theory. It was particularly influenced by the writings of Dickoff and James and their colleagues. The metatheory of Dickoff and James suggested a radically different view of practice theory than the scientific metatheory prevailing in the 1960s. They described a view of how theory can be developed and the nature of theory for a practice discipline (Dickoff and James, 1968; Dickoff, James, and Wiedenbach, 1968). Dickoff, James, and colleagues recognized the value-laden nature of theory in nursing and called for an explicit recognition and naming of the values toward which theory development was proceeding. Additionally, unlike the assumptions of traditional scientific theory, they acknowledged that theorizing around a valued outcome would never be complete. The inclusion of values within the structure of theory and the recognition that theory was more a flexible guide to practice provided a revolutionary view of empiric knowledge. The Dickoff and James approach to nursing metatheory, which was intensely discussed in the literature and at conferences, reflected a growing recognition that the nature and value of scientific-empiric theory for nursing was unclear. Nurses were required to question the nature of theory and the value of practice theory and to attempt a clearer concept of nursing practice.

Other approaches to developing empiric models and theories defining nursing as a practice discipline combined direct observations of nurses and their practice and systematizing insights derived from existing theories, models, and philosophies of nursing and other literature sources. Theoretic ideas developed in the 1960s and 1970s broadly defined nursing and named the phenomena central to nursing's domain of concern. These ideas shifted nursing away from a medical model of practice. They described how nursing functions to achieve a socially relevant purpose and specified the contextual variables important to the practice of nursing. A philosophic component in early nursing theories reflects central assumptions and value positions on which nursing rests. At the same time, early theories were characterized by a relatively functional view of nursing and health. They defined what nursing is, described the social purposes nursing serves, detailed how nurses function to realize these purposes, and defined the parameters and variables influencing illness and health processes.

For example, Callista Roy, Dorothea Orem, Virginia Henderson, and Hildegard Peplau focused on descriptions of illness and health—what nurses do to assist the person to move toward health. These theories present explanations of how nursing actions function in practice to enhance health and well-being. The functions described are theoretic in nature, in that they are conceptualized at a relatively abstract level. Nursing is viewed as a set of roles or functions, not as concrete technical procedures. These abstract ideas about nursing functions are woven into explanations of relationships between the nurse's roles and function and the theorist's idea of a desired nursing outcome related to health and well-being.

In the later 1970s and the 1980s there is a noticeable qualitative shift in theoretic ideas developed for the purpose of broadly defining nursing practice. Rather than reflect a functional perspective of the role of nursing in society, later theories tend to move to qualitative dimensions that characterize nursing's role as not what nurses do but as the essence of what nursing is. This shift offers potential for moving nursing from a context-dependent reactive position to a context-interactive proactive stance.

For example, both Jean Watson and Patricia Benner have developed theories of nursing that ground the essence of nursing in caring. They use theoretic reasoning that is derived from a deliberate philosophic stance that is explicit in their writings and from experience of the practice of nursing in many different contexts. The themes or patterns that characterize the essence of caring theory are those reflected in the actions, thoughts, values, and priorities of the practicing nurse.

The Development of Midrange Practice-Linked Theory

During the 1980s, Meleis (1987) brought into clear focus the need for nurses to develop substantive theory that provides a meaningful foundation for the development of nursing practice in relation to specific practice concepts. In accord with the observation of many practicing nurses, Meleis acknowledged the value of broad-scope theories in defining general parameters on which nursing function is based but emphasized that theory of a different type was required to give more specific guidance for nursing practice, a form of theory that, it turns out, would more closely align with the scientific-empiric pattern of knowing and knowledge. Meleis's plea also reflected the need for nursing to move away from its long-term discussions and debates about the nature of theory, knowledge, and the proper functions of nursing. She called on nurses to focus on developing substance in theory—that is, a focus on nursing concepts grounded in a practice context. Theory of this type is developed in concert with research questions directly linked to important practice problems. It avoids a focus on methodology for methodology's sake and shifts the focus to understanding nursing phenomena. Substantive theory can inform practice and lead to new practice approaches and factors that influence the outcomes desired in nursing practice.

Midrange theory tends to cluster around a concept of interest, such as social support, pain, grief, fatigue, or life transitions. Several nurse researcher-scholars may work in concert with practitioner-scholars to develop theory related to a substantive area of concern. Each theorist's perspective contributes to developing research, theory, and practice in the substantive area. Appendix B reviews selected examples of currently developing midrange theory in nursing.

OVERVIEW OF CONCEPTUAL THEMES IN NURSING THEORIES AND FRAMEWORKS

Many of the theoretic writings that proliferated during the 1960s and 1970s are still growing and changing. Table 2-1 presents a chronologic list of nurse theorists prior to 1990 who have produced broad theoretic conceptualiza-

TABLE 2-1 Chronology of Conceptual Models in Nursing (1952-1989)

Year of First Major Publication	Theorist	Key Emphasis
1952	Hildegard E. Peplau	Interpersonal process is maturing force for personality.
1960	Faye G. Abdellah Irene L. Beland Almeda Martin Ruth V. Matheney	Patient's problems determine nursing care.
1961	Ida Jean Orlando	Interpersonal process alleviates distress.
1964	Ernestine Wiedenbach	Helping process meets needs through art of individualizing care.
1966	Lydia E. Hall	Nursing care is person directed toward self-love.
1966	Joyce Travelbee	Meaning in illness determines how people respond.
1967	Myra E. Levine	Wholism is maintained by conserving integrity.
1970	Martha E. Rogers	Person-environment are energy fields that evolve negentropically.
1971	Dorothea E. Orem	Self-care maintains wholeness.
1971	Imogene M. King	Transactions provide a frame of reference toward goal setting.
1976	Callista Roy	Stimuli disrupt an adaptive system.
1976	Josephine G. Paterson Loretta T. Zderad	Nursing is an existential experience of nurturing.
1978	Madeleine M. Leininger	Caring is universal and varies transculturally.
1979	Jean Watson	Caring is moral ideal: mind-body-soul engagement with another.
1979	Margaret A. Newman	Disease is a clue to pre-existing life patterns.
1980	Dorothy E. Johnson	Subsystems exist in dynamic stability.
1981	Rosemarie Rizzo Parse	Indivisible beings and environment cocreate health.
1989	Patricia Benner and Judith Wrubel	Caring is central to the essence of nursing. It sets up what matters, enabling connection and concern. It creates possibility for mutual helpfulness.

tions or models of nursing. The table also includes our view of the key emphasis of each theorist's work. A more in-depth interpretive summary of the writings of each theorist listed in the table can be found in Appendix A. As you examine this table and the appendix, you might notice that, over time, the focus for these theoretic perspectives changed significantly. These changes paralleled changes in society. Systems theory had widespread acceptance in the biologic and social sciences during the 1960s, and its influence can be particularly noted in the work of Imogene King, Dorothy Johnson, Betty Neuman, and Callista Roy. The theories of Martha Rogers, Rosemarie Parse, and Margaret Newman reflect theoretic perspectives linked to modern physics that move beyond earlier system concepts of equilibrium.

Theorists continue to develop their ideas, and they often change their perspectives. These changes are linked to research findings when theories are used, peer critique, growth in the theorists' ideas, and changes in the social and political contexts within which nursing theories develop. Theorists whose perspective have changed considerably with successive publications include Callista Roy, Jean Watson, and Madeleine Leininger.

Theoretic ideas in nursing models and frameworks can also be grouped according to common traits or features. For example, Ernestine Wiedenbach and Ida Jean Orlando both focus on the importance of meeting patient needs. Although from different perspectives, Leininger and Watson both emphasize the concept of caring as a central focus for nursing. When various theoretic writings are grouped around common themes, central concepts or images for nursing are formed.

Four elements are widely recognized as common themes that can be found in most of nursing's theoretic literature: nursing, the person, society and environment, and health.

Nursing

In nursing's theoretic writings, nursing is generally represented as a helping process with a primary focus on interpersonal interactions between a nurse and another individual. This general idea does not clearly distinguish nursing from other helping disciplines, but it provides an important focus for deciding what kind of knowledge is needed in nursing practice. The interpersonal nature of nursing practice distinguishes nursing from medicine, in that medicine focuses on surgical and pharmacologic interventions, with interpersonal interactions secondary to these interventions. Within a medical model of nursing, the nurse's primary functions relate to medical assessment, diagnosis and treatment, and medication administration as delegated medical tasks. Within a nursing framework, when interpersonal interactions are primary; technical and medical functions support the primary interpersonal interactions.

Although different nurse authors present conceptualizations of the nature of nursing that are consistent with the idea of interpersonal interactions as a primary focus, there are important differences in their definitions and conceptualizations. For some, the direction of the interaction and the specific actions that are taken in achieving the goals of the interaction are largely defined by the person with whom the nurse interacts. The nurse's role in the interaction is primarily one of facilitating. When this view of the nature of nursing is incorporated into a framework or model, nursing is viewed as enabling the will and behavior of the person receiving care.

Other theoretic models present a view of the interpersonal process as either shared or initiated by the nurse. In this view, nursing processes and actions rest primarily on the nurse's initiative, knowledge, and approaches. The theoretic ideas that emerge from this view focus on nursing actions to reach the goal of the interaction.

Each of these perspectives is consistent with the practice of nursing in that nurses encounter some situations in which the client primarily directs the interaction and other situations in which the nurse is the initiator, and some nursing theories account for this diversity. The common significant thread is the primacy of human interaction in creating human health and wholeness. Table 2-2 describes the concept of nursing as reflected in the work of several nurse theorists.

The Person

All nursing frameworks and models include ideas about the general nature of human beings. The most consistent philosophic component of the idea of the person is the dimension of wholeness, or wholism. Although various conceptual frameworks may view the ill or diseased person as having problems with need fulfillment, integration, adaptation, role fulfillment, and so forth, the central impediment to health or healing is dealt with wholistically in various senses of the word.

The nature of wholism as a concept is difficult to address from the perspective of traditional Western philosophies that are grounded in reductionism. In the reductionist view of wholism, the whole is equal to the sum of the parts; interrelationships among parts are understood, and generalizations can be made about the whole (Newman, 1979). Western culture is located within this view, and nurses, like others in this culture, have learned to think about parts of lives, parts of bodies, and parts of human experiences.

In a purer sense more consistent with Eastern traditions, wholism means that the whole is greater than the sum of the parts. The whole cannot be reduced to parts without losing something in the process. Martha Rogers, Margaret Newman, Joyce Travelbee, and Patricia Benner are examples of nurse scholars whose work reflects a view that the individual is different from and greater than the sum of the parts. Other nursing theorists explicitly or implicitly hold that wholism is equal to the sum of parts, assuming the

TABLE 2-2 Theoretic Ideas About Nursing

Author	Concepts of Nursing
Hildegard Peplau (1952)	Nursing is a significant therapeutic interpersonal process. The interpersonal process is a maturing force and educative instrument for both nurse and client. Self-knowledge in the context of the interpersonal interaction is essential to understanding the client and reaching resolution of the problem. There are four sequential phases of the interpersonal process: (1) orientation, (2) identification, (3) exploitation, and (4) resolution.
Ida Jean Orlando (1961)	Nursing is a process of interaction with an ill individual to meet an immediate need. The nursing situation consists of (1) the person's behavior, (2) the nurse's reaction, and (3) nursing action appropriate to the person's need. The nurse is accountable to the individual receiving care.
Ernestine Wiedenbach (1964)	There are three components of nursing: (1) identification of a person's need for help, (2) ministration of the help needed, and (3) validation that the help provided was indeed helpful. The nursing process begins with an activating situation that arouses the nurse's consciousness. Clinical nursing has four components: philosophy, purpose, practice, and art.
Myra Levine (1967)	Nursing care is both supportive and therapeutic. Supportive interventions are designed to maintain a state of wholeness as consistently as possible with failing adaptation. Therapeutic interventions are designed to promote adaptation that contributes to health and restoration of health. All nursing actions are based on conservation of energy, structural integrity, personal integrity, and social integrity.
Jean Watson (1979)	Nursing is a human science and an art that is based on the moral ideal and value of caring. There are 10 carative factors that constitute the knowledge and practice of human care nursing. The context of nursing is humanitarian and metaphysic; the goal of nursing is to gain a higher degree of harmony in mind, body, and soul, which leads to self-knowledge, self-reverence, self-healing, and self-care.

individual is a system with biologic, sociologic, and psychologic components. Although not consistent with wholism in its purest sense, there is still a strong commitment to the idea that all components of the individual need to be considered (Flaskerud and Halloran, 1980). Table 2-3 describes the concept of person as reflected in the work of several nurse theorists.

TABLE 2-3   Theoretic Ideas About the Person

Author	Concepts of Person
Joyce Travelbee (1966)	A single human being, family, or community whose illness experience has unique meaning.
Virginia Henderson (1966)	Mind and body are inseparable. No two individuals are alike; each is unique. The individual's basic needs are reflected in 14 components of basic nursing care.
Martha Rogers (1970)	Unitary human being is viewed as an energy field, the boundaries of which extend beyond the discernible mass of the human body. There are five unifying assumptions about the life process: (1) unified wholeness, (2) openness, (3) unidirectionality, (4) pattern and organization, and (5) sentience.
Dorothea Orem (1971)	The individual is an integrated whole composed of an internal physical, psychologic, and social nature with varying degrees of self-care ability.
Imogene King (1971)	Individuals are viewed as (1) reacting beings, (2) time-oriented beings, and (3) social beings, with the ability to perceive, think, feel, choose, set goals, and make decisions.
Patricia Benner and Judith Wrubel (1989)	The person is a self-interpreting being engaged in the world. Engagement is possible because of the human capacities of embodied intelligence, culturally acquired meanings, concern, and direct involvement in or grasp of a situation.

Society and Environment

The concept of society and environment is central to the discipline of nursing and is reflected across conceptual frameworks, although these ideas are not addressed as explicitly in some writings as in others. Several nursing frameworks include a concept of society or culture and view it as a critical interacting force shaping the individual (Table 2-4). The environment was central for Nightingale in formulating her concept of nursing. Nightingale believed that the primary focus for nursing was to alter the physical environment to place the human body in the best possible condition for the reparative processes of nature to occur. Several conceptual models de-emphasize environment per se or view it as encompassed within a concept of society, sometimes using the word *society* to include environment. However, the concept of environment has reemerged as a significant one. Martha Rogers and theorists who build on her ideas focus on a concept of environment as indistinguishable (except conceptually) from the concept of person. Most other conceptual frameworks separate person from

TABLE 2-4 Theoretic Ideas About Society and Environment

Author	Concepts of Society and Environment
Florence Nightingale (1860)	Environment is the central concept. It is viewed as all external conditions and influences that affect life and the development of the organism. The major emphasis is on warmth, effluvia (odors), noise, and light.
Joyce Travelbee (1966)	Environment is the context in which human-to-human relatedness or rapport is established.
Myra Levine (1967)	Society is viewed as the total environment of the individual, including family, significant others, and the nurse.
Callista Roy (1976)	Environment constantly interacts with the individual and determines, in part, adaptation level. Stimuli originate in the environment.
Margaret Newman (1986)	Environment and person form a unitary pattern that is reflected in movement-space-time patterns of consciousness. Environment encompasses the total situation and is one with the person; environment includes the universe.

environment, implying boundaries that define the two. As with the concept of person, environmental concepts vary, but they appear across conceptual frameworks.

Health

The concept of health is typically identified as the goal of nursing. Nightingale stated that "the same laws of health or of nursing, for in reality they are the same, obtain among the well as among the sick" (Nightingale, 1969, p. 9), implying health as a state of order within natural laws. Contemporary nursing models are remarkably congruent with this early conceptualization. Some theories and models are based on a conceptualization of a health-illness continuum, and nursing's purpose is to assist the ill client to achieve the highest possible degree of health. Other nurse authors view the concept of health as something more than, or different from, the absence of disease. Health exists independently from illness or disease. In these views, it is a dynamic process that changes with time and varies with life circumstances. Some authors view the health process as interdependent with circumstances of the environment, whereas others view the health process as something that originates with the individual (Smith, 1983).

In an attempt to deal more specifically with ideas related to health, several nurse authors avoid using the terms *health* and *illness*. An example is Levine's

TABLE 2-5   Theoretic Ideas About Health

Author	Terms Related to Health
Lydia Hall (1966)	Self-actualization, self-love
Virginia Henderson (1966)	Independent function
Myra Levine (1967)	Maintaining wholism/conservation
Dorothea Orem (1971)	Self-care agency
Josephine Paterson and Loretta Zderad (1976)	Authentic awareness
Callista Roy (1976)	Continual adaptation
Margaret Newman (1986)	Expanding consciousness
Patricia Jones and Afaf I. Meleis (1993)	Empowerment

(1967) use of the term *conserving wholism*. This concept directs nurses to focus on the totality of a person's situation rather than on the typical parameters that have come to be commonly known as health. Table 2-5 identifies some of the terms that nurses have used in constructing their theoretic ideas about health. These terms suggest ideas that more specifically reflect nursing's concerns and de-emphasize the focus on disease or illness.

THE CONTEXTS OF KNOWLEDGE DEVELOPMENT

Nursing history has created, and continues to create, specific circumstances and contexts that influence the development of knowledge. They can be considered as belonging to or affecting the individual, the profession, and society. Table 2-6 lists values and resources that continue to influence the development of knowledge in nursing.

Values

Individual values include an individual's commitment, personal philosophy, motives, beliefs, and priorities. Professional values are beliefs and ideologies that are generally held in common by members of the profession and are used to guide professional action. They are expressed in formal statements issued by professional groups in the form of codes, standards of practice, and ethical theory and are also reflected in repeated themes that occur in the literature and in the collective actions taken by professional organizations.

Societal values are ideologies expressed through societal choices, sanctions, and mores during a given period in history. When individual, professional, and societal values are basically congruent, there is relative stability, and new insights tend to build on what is already established as knowledge in the discipline. When individual, professional, or societal values

TABLE 2-6 Values and Resources That Influence Theory Development

Source of Influence	Examples of Specific Factors
Values	
Individual	Commitment to the discipline
	Philosophy of nursing
	Motives
	Worldview or philosophy
	Priorities for action
Professional	Commitment to development of knowledge
	Code of ethics
	Standards for practice
	Standards for protecting participants
	Willingness to challenge social traditions
	Priorities for allocating resources
Society	Cultural mores
	Ethical codes
	Priorities for allocating resources
Resources	
Individual	Cognitive style
	Intellectual ability
	Personality
	Lifestyle and setting
	Educational background
	Life experience
	Economic power
Professional	Educational requirements for members
	Body of literature and communication style
	Methodologies and instrumentation
	Practice traditions
	Educational, economic, and political group profile
Society	Settings for practice, education, and research
	Funding for the discipline's activities
	Material resources

are in conflict, the potential exists for creating fundamental change in knowledge and in practice.

Resources

Resources can also be viewed as individual, professional, and societal. Individual resources include the natural and acquired talents shared among members of the discipline, including cognitive style, intellectual abilities, life circumstances, and educational preparation. The collective membership of the discipline forms the professional resources that support ongoing theory development. Examples of professional resources include a growing body of literature and practice traditions, the ability to communicate these among members of the profession, the educational attainments of members of the profession and the nature of their education, and methodologies and instrumentation available for theory development.

Societal resources are those circumstances, materials, space, and funds acquired by the profession from the society at large. Acquisition of societal resources depends on features of the society and the profession. For example, political influence is required to obtain funds, materials, and space to carry out the activities of the discipline. If the political system of society reflects priorities other than those that concern nursing, societal resources are less available to nursing than to other groups that reflect those priorities.

The problem of allocating resources illustrates the circular relationship between resources and values. Politics involves value decisions about who does and does not deserve the resources of society. If, as the course of history shows, women scientists are consistently provided limited or no societal resources, the ability of women to influence value decisions is lessened. Nursing is a group comprised mostly of women (a professional resource) within a societal context that devalues women as scientists. This fact influences the profession's ability to exert influence on society at large and gain access to resources. The contemporary women's movement has created a stimulus for recognizing societal restrictions on nursing as a sex-segregated occupation and the effects of systematic oppression on nurses and nursing (Greenleaf, 1980; Roberts, 1983). Feminist theory, which shares many of the traits of nursing theory, provides a perspective for changing social values and shifting social resources. Feminism places on society an urgent demand for a values transformation that is consistent with nursing's vision of health, the health care system, and nursing (Chinn and Wheeler, 1985). As women's experience is increasingly valued as a resource for developing knowledge, the resulting values conflict with traditional views, and the new values will open avenues for change.

Table 2-6 is intended to help you think about how, for example, your motives for becoming a nurse or changing your educational credentials and your given personality characteristics will influence your contributions to knowledge development within nursing, or, in the professional category, how you think nursing's collective practice traditions and willingness to challenge traditions influence knowledge development. Why, within the societal category, is funding for important nursing activities limited? How successful will nursing be in attending to a broad conceptualization of knowing when scientific knowledge is still largely held to be most valuable? We hope you will use the table to examine the significance of values and resources to question present-day practices in knowledge development.

CONCLUSION

In this chapter, we have presented an overview of the history from which our nursing knowledge evolves. The values and resources that influence knowledge development are rooted in history and determine how knowledge in nursing is seen and how it develops. The history, values, and resources of nursing have been influenced by cultural and societal circumstances that closely parallel the status and role of women. As early theorists in nursing developed a sense of community and scholarship, they expressed differences and commonalities that have influenced more recent theoretic developments. A perspective of history and an understanding of the values and resources affecting the development of theory make it possible to refine understandings of what knowledge is.

Reference List

Abdellah FG, Belard IL, Norton A, and Mathers, RV: *Patient-centered approaches to nursing,* New York, 1960, Macmillan.

Abdellah FG: The nature of nursing science, *Nurs Res* 18:390, 1969.

Achterberg J: *Woman as healer,* Boston, 1991, Shambhala.

Aikins CA: Teaching ethics in hospital schools, *Trained Nurs & Hosp Rev* 54:135, 1915.

Ashley J: *Hospitals, paternalism, and the role of the nurse,* New York, 1976, Teachers College Press.

Barnard KE, Neal MV: Maternal-child nursing research: review of the past and strategies for the future, *Nurs Res* 26, 193-200.

Benner P, Wrubel J: *The primacy of caring: stress and coping in health and illness,* Menlo Park, Calif, 1989, Addison Wesley.

Bixler GK, Bixler RW: The professional status of nursing, *Am J Nurs* 45:730, 1945.

Brigh M: We cannot afford to hurry: training within industry applied to nursing, *Am J Nurs* 44:223, 1944.

Burgess ME: A plan for nursing care, *Am J Nurs* 41:215, 1941.

Changes in nursing practice, *Am J Nurs* 47:665, 1947.

Chinn PL, Wheeler CE: Feminism and nursing, *Nurs Outlook* 33:74, 1985.

Christy TE: Portrait of a leader, *Nurs Outlook* 6:72, 1969.

Conrad ME: What is expert nursing care? *Am J Nurs* 47:162, 1947.

Dennis KE, Prescott PA: Florence Nightingale: yesterday, today, and tomorrow, *Adv Nurs Sci* 7(2):66, 1985.

De Witt K: Specialities in nursing, *Am J Nurs* 1:14, 1900-1901.

Dickoff J, James P: A theory of theories: a position paper, *Nurs Res* 17:197, 1968.

Dickoff J, James P: Clarity to what end? *Nurs Res* 20:499, 1971.

Dickoff J, James P, Wiedenbach E: Theory in a practice discipline. Part 1: practice-oriented theory, *Nurs Res* 17:415, 1968.

Drake A: How the patient judges nursing, *Trained Nurs & Hosp Rev* 93:135, 1934.

Ellis R: Commentary on "Toward a clearer understanding of the concept of nursing theory," *Nurs Res* 20:493, 1971.

Flaskerud JH, Halloran EJ: Areas of agreement in nursing theory development, *Adv Nurs Sci* 3(1):1, 1980.

Folta JR: Obsfucation or clarification: a reaction to Walker's concept of nursing theory, *Nurs Res* 20:196, 1971.

Garesche EF: Professional honor, *Am J Nurs* 27:901, 1927.

Greenleaf NP: Sex-segregated occupations: relevance for nursing, *Adv Nurs Sci* 2(3):23, 1980.

Gregg A: An independent estimate of nursing in our times, *Am J Nurs* 40:735, 1940.

Hall LE: A center for nursing, *Nurs Outlook* 11:805, 1963.

Hall LE: Nursing: what is it? *Can Nurs* 60:150, 1964.

Hall LE: Another view of nursing care and quality. In Straub KM, Parker KS, editors: *Continuity in patient care: the role of nursing,* Washington, DC, 1966, Catholic University Press.

Hardy ME: Perspectives on nursing theory, *Adv Nurs Sci* 1(1):37, 1978.

Henderson V: The nature of nursing, *Am J Nurs* 64:62, 1964.

Henderson V: *The nature of nursing,* New York, 1966, Macmillan.

Hughes L: The public image of the nurse, *Adv Nurs Sci* 2(3):55, 1980.

Johnson DE: Today's action will determine tomorrow's nursing, *Nurs Outlook* 13:38, 1965.

Johnson DE: The behavioral system model for nursing. In Riehl JP, Roy SC, editors: *Conceptual models for nursing practice,* ed 2, New York, 1980, Appleton-Century-Crofts.

Johnson PE: What should ethics teach? *Am J Nurs* 28:1084, 1928.

Jones PS, Meleis, AI: Health is empowerment. *Adv Nurs Sci* 15(3):114, 1993.

Kalisch PA, Kalisch BJ: *The advance of American nursing,* Boston, 1978, Little, Brown.

Kelly LY, Joel LA: *The nursing experience: trends, challenges and transitions,* ed 3, New York, 1996. McGraw-Hill.

King IM: *Toward a theory for nursing: general concepts of human behavior,* New York, 1971, John Wiley.

Leininger MM: Doctoral programs for nurses: trends, questions, and projected plans, *Nurs Res* 25:201, 1976.

Leininger MM: *Transcultural nursing: concepts, theories and practices,* New York, 1978, John Wiley.

Levine ME: The four conservation principles of nursing, *Nurs Forum* 6:93, 1967.

Lovell MC: The politics of medical deception: challenging the trajectory of history, *Adv Nurs Sci* 2(3), 73, 1980.

Meade AB: Training the senses in clinical observation, *Trained Nurs & Hosp Rev* 97:540, 1936.

Meleis AI: Revisions in knowledge development: a passion for substance, *Sch Inq Nurs Pract* 1:5, 1987.

Melosh B: *The physician's hand: work culture and conflict in American nursing,* Philadelphia, 1982, Temple University Press.

Mossman LC: The place of beauty in life, *Trained Nurs & Hosp Rev* 81:318, 1923.

Mountin JW: Nursing: a critical analysis, *Am J Nurs* 43:29, 1943.

Newman MA: *Theory development in nursing,* Philadelphia, 1979, FA Davis.

Newman MA: *Health as expanding consciousness,* St Louis, 1986, Mosby–Year Book.

Nightingale F: *Notes on Nursing: what it is and what it is not,* New York, 1969, Dover (originally published in 1860).

Nightingale F: *Cassandra,* New York, 1979, Feminist Press (originally published in 1852).

Noble GE: The spirit of nursing, *Am J Nurs* 40:161, 1940.

Oettinger KB: Toward inner freedom, *Am J Nurs* 39:1224, 1939.

Orem DE: *Nursing: concepts of practice,* New York, 1971, McGraw-Hill.

Orlando IJ: *The dynamic nurse-patient relationship: function, process, and principles,* New York, 1961, GP Putnam's (republished in 1990 by the National League for Nursing).

Parse RR: *Man-living-health: a theory of nursing,* New York, 1981, John Wiley.

Paterson JG, Zderad LT: *Humanistic nursing,* New York, 1976, John Wiley (republished in 1988 by the National League for Nursing).

Peplau HE: *Interpersonal relations in nursing,* New York, 1952, GP Putnam's.

Pfefferkorn F: What of nursing field studies? *Am J Nurs* 33:258, 1933.

Reverby SM: *Ordered to care: the dilemma of American nursing, 1850-1945,* Cambridge, 1987, Cambridge University Press.

Riddles AR: The force of example, *Trained Nurs & Hosp Rev* 80:27, 1928.

Roberts SJ: Oppressed group behavior: implications for nursing, *Adv Nurs Sci* 5(4):21, 1983.

Rogers ME: *An introduction to the theoretical basis of nursing,* Philadelphia, 1970, FA Davis.

Roy C: *Introduction to nursing: an adaptation model,* Englewood Cliffs, NJ, 1976, Prentice-Hall.

Sanger M: *Margaret Sanger, an autobiography,* New York, 1971, Dover (originally published in 1938 by WW Norton).

Silverstein NG: Lillian Wald at Henry Street, 1893-1895, *Adv Nurs Sci* 7(2):1, 1985.

Simpson LF: The psychology of nursing, *Trained Nurs & Hosp Rev* 52:133, 1914.

Smith JA: *The idea of health: implications for the nursing professional,* New York, 1983, Teachers College Press.

Tooley SA: *The life of Florence Nightingale,* New York, 1905, Macmillan.

Travelbee J: *Interpersonal aspects of nursing,* Philadelphia, 1966, FA Davis.

Wald L: *The house on Henry Street,* New York, 1971, Dover (originally published in 1915 by Holt, Rinehart, & Winston).

Walker LO: Toward a clearer understanding of the concept of nursing theory, *Nurs Res* 20:428, 1971.

Warnshius FC: The future of medicine and nursing: the ideal to be sought, *Am J Nurs* 26:123, 1926.

Watson J: *Nursing: the philosophy and science of caring,* Boston, 1979, Little, Brown (republished in 1988 by the National League for Nursing).

Whall AL: Congruence between existing theories of family functioning and nursing theories, *Adv Nurs Sci* 3(1):59, 1980.

Wheeler CE: The *American Journal of Nursing* and the socialization of a profession, *Adv Nurs Sci* 7:20, 1985.

Wiedenbach E: *Clinical nursing: a helping art,* New York, 1964, Springer.

Woodham-Smith C: *Florence Nightingale: 1820-1910,* New York, 1983, Atheneum.

Wooldridge PJ: Meta-theories of nursing: a commentary on Dr. Walker's article, *Nurs Res* 20:494, 1971.

Worcester A: Is nursing really a profession? *Am J Nurs* 2:908, 1902.

Chapter 3

Empiric Knowledge Development: Explaining and Structuring

Looking at human behavior is like running into a cloud whose origins and direction is unknown. You can see the cloud, dynamic and three dimensional, but when you reach out to grab a handful to test you come away with nothing visible but a clenched fist. You may be buffeted by the forces within the cloud that moves on, still visible and dynamic and still three dimensional and you think "I can see the cloud, I can feel the forces it contains, but how do I study it when it refuses to lend itself to anything more than a fleeting encounter?"

Marjorie R. Wright (1966, p. 244)

In this chapter we focus on methods for explaining and structuring empiric phenomena. Figure 3-1 shows the empiric quadrant of our model for nursing knowledge development, highlighting the role of explaining and structuring ideas into formal expressions such as theories and models. Theories and models in turn become shared as empiric knowledge in the discipline and serve to enable scientific competence in practice.

Two processes are involved in explaining and structuring empiric phenomena: (1) creating conceptual meaning and (2) structuring and contextualizing theory. In this chapter we focus on theory; however, there are other empiric knowledge forms such as conceptual models or frameworks, principles, and rich descriptions of empiric phenomena. Theory is the most formal, most highly structured of the empiric knowledge forms.

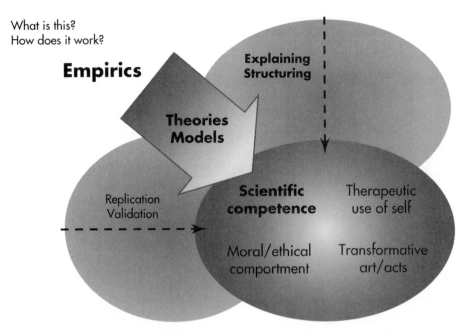

FIGURE 3-1 The empiric pattern of knowing: explaining and structuring empiric phenomena to create formal expressions of empiric knowledge and to develop scientific competence.

Conceptual frameworks, models, and descriptions also require well-developed conceptual meaning and sufficient structure to adequately represent the relationships within their scope.

WHAT IS EMPIRIC THEORY?

The idea of theory carries varying conceptualizations within and outside the discipline of nursing. Defining *theory* is not easy, and ultimately most people accept an arbitrary meaning. Just when a definition seems firm, another idea surfaces that must be integrated into the definition. Theory has common, everyday connotations apparent in such phrases as "I have a theory about that" or "my theory is." These usages imply that theory is an idea or feeling or that it explains something. In this book, we use a definition that is consistent with the more everyday meanings of theory as a collection of ideas or explanatory hunches. But our definition goes beyond this to a characterization of theory as something deliberately designed for a specific purpose.

Beliefs about the nature of theory arise in part from the various fields of inquiry from which nursing knowledge is developed. Some nursing theorists come from traditions in which the ideal of theory is logically linked sets of confirmed hypotheses. Others view theory as loosely connected hypothetic conjectures. Still others think of theory as philosophically based sets of beliefs and values about human nature and action. As a result, the nursing literature contains varying definitions for *theory*, but this diversity serves to stimulate further understanding and development of theory. Four definitions in the nursing literature emphasize important dimensions of theory.

1. A logically interconnected set of confirmed hypotheses (McKay, 1969). This definition implies a specific form of expression based on rules of logic. It also requires that the hypotheses are tested and confirmed by using methods of research to qualify as a theory.
2. A conceptual system or framework invented to some purpose (Dickoff and James, 1968). In this definition, the purpose for which a theory is created is emphasized. The term *invented* implies a creative process.
3. An imaginative grouping of knowledge, ideas, and experience that are represented symbolically and seek to illuminate a given phenomenon (Watson, 1985). Here creativity is again emphasized, but the purpose for which theory is created shifts away from a specific purpose to the aim of enhancing understanding of a given phenomenon.
4. Conceptual and pragmatic principles forming a general frame of reference for a field of inquiry (Ellis, 1968). This definition implies that theory provides a philosophic view that guides inquiry in a discipline and also that theory serves a pragmatic or practical purpose for the discipline.

From our perspective, all theory comprises a creative and rigorous structuring of ideas. The ideas are structured as concepts that are represented by word symbols. For theory to project a systematic view of phenomena, the concepts contained within the theory must be conveyed within relationship statements and defined within the context of the theory. The theorist creates a language and structure that impart to theory its systematic nature. Theory is purposive; theorists create theory for some reason. The purpose may take many forms. Theory is tentative and thus is grounded in assumptions, value choices, and the creative and imaginative judgment of the theorist. Therefore, our definition of theory is:

> **theory** A creative and rigorous structuring of ideas that projects a tentative, purposeful, and systematic view of phenomena.

The word *creative* underscores the role of human imagination and vision in the development and expression of theory. It does not mean that "anything goes" or that theory is improvised. Creative processes required to develop theory are also rigorous, systematic, and disciplined, yielding a well-developed conception that also bears the mark of the creator. In our view, theoretic statements are tentative, open to revision as new evidence and new insights emerge. The statements are developed toward some purpose or within a specific context. Our definition does not require that a hypothesis be tested before the statements can be considered as theory. Ideas that the creator systematically develops based on experience and observation can be considered as theory prior to formal testing.

Given our definition, it is possible to analyze how theory differs from related terms such as *science, philosophy, paradigm,* and *model.* Like the word *theory,* these terms are highly abstract and have multiple meanings. To resolve differences between similar yet different terms such as *theoretic framework* and *theory,* definitions of both can be created. It is possible to arrive at definitions for different terms that are alike, and it is equally possible that definitions for the same term will reflect fundamental differences in meaning. But within any context, abstract terms need to be defined to convey how each is being used within that context. Our definitions of several related terms for the context of this book are shown in Table 3-1. The definitions of related terms—like our definition of *theory*—may not be universally accepted, but we believe that they are reasonable and reflect common meanings.

CREATING CONCEPTUAL MEANING

Creating conceptual meaning is a theory-building approach that depends on mental processes. This means that mental constructions or ideas are used to represent experience. What is mentally constructed is expressed in words. The process of creating conceptual meaning assumes common yet unique human experiences and shared meaning among people. At the same time, it is a process that assumes that a person's own subjective construction of reality is more accessible than anything else.

The process of creating conceptual meaning brings dimensions of meaning to a conscious, communicable awareness. Because of the limits of language, the process of creating conceptual meaning also makes it possible to identify the limits of conveying empirical meaning. Despite its limitations, language is a powerful tool that shapes perceptions and shapes meaning (Müller & Dzurec, 1993). If someone is called clever, that person begins to form an awareness of self that may be new. At the same time, the word *clever* may not adequately express the rich inner experiences and instead trivialize what is experienced within. If the word represents a desired value, the description given contributes positively to self-awareness.

TABLE 3-1 Conceptual Definitions of Terms Related to the Concept of Theory

Term	Definition
Science	An approach to the generation of empiric knowledge that relies on accessible sensory experience to create knowledge and to form understanding. The term also refers to the results of using systematic methods of empirics. The process involves critical and logical thought; the results yield the facts, theories, and descriptions of the discipline. Natural science assumes that the scientist and the object of study are separate and that what is being studied is governed by laws and rules that do not vary. Human science approaches take into account the thinking, feeling, and intentional characteristics of human nature and assumes that the scientist influences the reality that is studied.
Philosophy	A form of disciplined inquiry that discerns the nature of reality and of knowledge and knowing, ways of discerning reality, and principles of value. Philosophy relies on logic and reasoning, rather than empiric evidence, to create knowledge.
Research	An application of formalized methods of obtaining reliable and valid knowledge about empiric experience.
Fact	That which is generally held to be an empirically verifiable object, property, or event, meaning that the phenomenon is experienced and named consistently and similarly by others given a similar context.
Model	A symbolic representation of an empiric experience in the form of words, pictorial or graphic diagrams, mathematic notations, or physical material (such as a model airplane).
Theoretical or conceptual framework	A logical grouping of related concepts or theories, usually created to draw several different aspects together that are relevant to a complex situation, such as a practice setting or an educational program.
Paradigm	A worldview or ideology. A paradigm implies standards or criteria for assigning value or worth to both the processes and the products of a discipline, as well as for the methods of knowledge development within a discipline.

Although creating conceptual meaning provides a foundation for developing theory and is a logical starting point for theory development, it does not necessarily have to be accomplished first. It is a process that can be done by the beginning and advanced scholar and by the novice and expert practitioner. As the term for this process implies, we believe that conceptual meaning is something that is created. It does not exist as an "out there" reality to be objectively discovered. Rather, it is deliberately formed from experience. Although this process is critical to all theory development, it is often overlooked (Norris, 1982). Most theorists provide definitions of terms used within theory, but forming word definitions is not the same as creating meaning. Conceptual meaning conveys thoughts, feelings, and ideas that reflect the human experience of the concept.

What Is a Concept?

We define the term *concept* as a complex mental formulation of experience. By "experience," we mean perceptions of the world—objects, other people, visual images, color, movement, sounds, behavior, interactions—the totality of what is perceived. Experience is considered empiric when it can be symbolically shared and verified by others with sensory evidence. Three sources of experience interact to form the meaning of the idea: (1) the word or other symbolic label, (2) the thing itself (object, property, or event), and (3) feelings, values, and attitudes associated with the word and with the perception of the thing.

Conceptual meaning is created by considering all three sources of experiences related to the concept: the word, the thing itself, and the associated feelings. The same word may be used to represent more than one phenomenon. For example, the word *cup* may be used to represent several different kinds of objects or ideas. Each use of the word carries with it different perceptions. If the object is a fancy teacup, a very different mental image forms than if the object is the cup into which a golf ball falls on a putting green. The word *love,* a more abstract concept, can be used to describe a feeling toward a parent, child, pet, car, job, friend, or intimate partner, with each use implying an essentially different but related feeling.

All concepts can be located on a continuum from the empiric (more directly experienced) to the abstract (more mentally constructed) (Jacox, 1974; Kaplan, 1964). In one sense, all concepts are both empiric and abstract. They are empiric because they are formed from encounters with perceptible reality. They are abstract because they are cognitive representations of what is perceptually experienced. Concepts differ in their relationship to perceptible reality. Some concepts are formed from very direct experiences with reality, whereas others are formed from indirect experiences. Figure 3-2 illustrates this continuum. Relatively empiric concepts are ideas that are formed from direct observations of objects, properties, or events. As concepts become more abstract, they can be experienced only indirectly. The most abstract concepts encompass a complex network of subconcepts that can only be inferred.

The most concrete empiric concepts have direct forms of measurement. Concepts formed about objects such as a cup or properties such as hot are examples of highly empiric concepts because the object or property that represents the idea (empiric indicator) can be directly experienced through

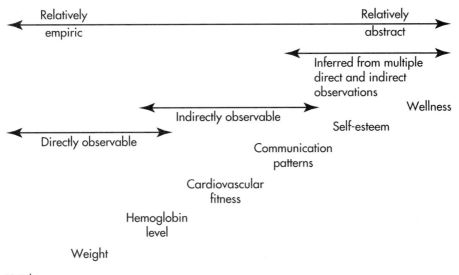

FIGURE 3-2 Example of continuum of empiric abstraction.

the senses. A relatively empiric property such as biologic sex can also be observed directly by noting the primary and secondary sexual characteristics that identify a person as male or female or, more precisely, by identifying chromosomal patterns. Properties such as height and weight can be measured with standardized instruments.

As concepts become more abstract, their reality basis and their empiric indicators become less concrete and less directly measurable. Assessment of an abstract concept depends increasingly on indirect means. Although an indirect assessment or observation is different from direct measurement, it is considered a reasonable indicator of the concept. Hemoglobin level is representative of a concept that cannot be directly observed but can be indirectly seen with the aid of laboratory instruments. This type of measurement depends on more complex and less direct forms of instrumentation.

Cardiovascular fitness is an example of a concept that is midrange on the empiric-abstract continuum. Concepts increase in complexity in this range, and several empiric indicators must be assessed. Because no object such as cardiovascular fitness exists, a definition is required if we are to know what it is. Even though definitions for less empirically based concepts are thoughtfully formulated, they are arbitrary because many different definitions could be chosen. As concepts become increasingly abstract, definitions become more dependent on the theoretic meaning of the concept and the purpose for defining it.

Self-esteem is an example of a highly abstract concept for which there are no direct measures. The instruments or tools that are developed to assess self-esteem depend on theoretic definitions serving a specific purpose and are built on multiple behavioral responses that experts agree are associated with that concept. Ideas about these responses may be derived from a theory or from concept clarification. Each behavioral trait contained in the tool can be considered as a partial indicator of self-esteem. When the composite behaviors are built into an assessment tool, it is usually a more adequate indicator for the abstract concept than any one behavior taken alone. The composite score obtained from the tool is then considered to be a measurement constructed as an empiric indicator.

Highly abstract concepts are sometimes called *constructs*. Constructs are the most complex type of concept on the empiric-abstract continuum. These concepts include ideas with a reality base so abstract that it is constructed from multiple sources of direct and indirect evidence. An example of a construct is wellness. Although the idea of wellness exists, it cannot be directly observed. Figure 3-1 illustrates the idea that highly abstract concepts are constructed from other concepts. All concepts shown on the continuum (as well as others) can be included in the concept of wellness.

Some abstract concepts have little meaning outside the context of a theory. For example, Levine (1967) coined the word *trophicogenic* to mean "nurse-induced illness." Rogers (1970) discussed three "principles of homeodynamics." Rogers's term *homeodynamics* is a combination of the Latin root word *homeo,* meaning "similar to" or "like," and the common English term *dynamics,* meaning "pattern of change or growth." The reader can infer the meaning "change processes" for the term *homeodynamics,* which is consistent with Rogers's intent.

Abstract concepts may also acquire additional meaning through gradual transfer into common language usage. Freud's concept of ego is an example. The word *ego* once had no common meaning outside Freud's theory, but today, with gradual changes in its meaning and broad usage outside the theory, everyone knows the meaning of "a big ego."

Although it is usually not possible to identify precisely where concepts fit on an empiric-abstract continuum, it is important to understand that concepts vary in the degree to which they are connected to empiric reality and the extent to which their meaning is mentally constructed. When you begin to study an abstract concept, it is natural to wonder why it is difficult to grasp the meaning of the term and understand all that is conveyed by the concept.

A single phenomenon can also be represented by several different words. Each word conveys a slightly different meaning, often nuances that relate to socially derived value meanings. For example, the words *car, Rolls,* and *hot wheels* can all refer to one thing—an automobile. Using any of these words to describe the object conveys more about the perspective or value of the person using the word than it does about the object itself. As the words acquire contextual and value meanings, they shift further toward the abstract.

Feelings, values, and attitudes are inner processes that are associated with experiences and words. For example, the word *mother* carries feelings, values, and attitudes that form in human experience with an actual person. Varying experiences with mother (the person) account for a range of feelings that different people associate with the word *mother.* At the same time, human meaning of the concept mother is formed from cultural and societal heritages that all people of a culture share, regardless of individual experiences in early childhood. A concept like mother, which can carry specific or highly complex meanings, moves from one end to the other in levels of abstraction, depending on the context of usage.

Many nursing concepts are highly abstract. Although theory and other common forms of empiric knowledge such as models, frameworks, and descriptions incorporate and depend on highly empiric facts, it is not factually based concepts that nursing theory reflects. Box 3-1 contains an exercise that may be useful in understanding the challenges involved in exploring and creating conceptual meaning.

Methods for Creating Conceptual Meaning

Creating conceptual meaning produces a tentative definition of the concept and a set of tentative criteria for determining if the concept exists in a particular situation. We use the word *tentative* because both the definition and the criteria can be revised. The term *tentative* does not mean that anything goes or that any definition that suits the author will do. This process is a deliberative, disciplined activity. The person who is creating meaning draws on many information sources, examines many possible dimensions of meaning, and presents ideas so that they can be tested and challenged in the light of the purposes for which the concept is being clarified.

There are various methods for creating conceptual meaning. Norris (1982) described several methods for concept clarification. Walker and Avant (1995) described a method of concept analysis based on the work of Wilson (1963). Morse (1995) described methods of concept development and analysis that draw on qualitative and quantitative research approaches to

Box 3-1

An Exercise in Creating a Concept and Exploring Various Complex Dimensions of Concepts

Close your eyes and imagine a "cup." Take a few minutes to notice what the cup is like. Notice what feelings are associated with it. Notice where it is and any other features of context. You might want to make a mental or written note when you open your eyes.

Congratulations! Well, maybe this wasn't such an unusual feat but you did create a concept.

If you haven't already done so, write a definition of *cup* based on what you saw.

Now, examine the definition. Did your cup have a handle? Did it have a hard surface that you described? Was it decorated? Was there anything in it? Did you smell anything?

Did you describe a cup that is used for drinking something? If you did (which we are betting on!), think about as many other images of "cup" as you can.

What did you come up with?

Did you think of the cup on a golfing green? A cup of a woman's brassiere? Did you think of anything like a "cup of cheer"? There is an image associated with that sort of cup, but can you see it and touch it? No, but you could recognize it.

Place your cup images on an empiric-abstract continuum.

A coffee type of cup is more empirically based (we can see and touch that!), but a cup of cheer is much more abstract. Remember Aunt Gracie who dutifully offered that wedding toast to a nephew she really didn't like much? She went through the motions, but did she mean it? Would her intention influence your use of the phrase "cup of cheer" to describe her action?

What did you notice about context when you described your initial cup image? When you take your original cup image and insert it into another context, what do you notice?

Would you imagine a group of groggy campers around a morning campfire sipping coffee from bone china cups on dainty saucers? Probably not, but these are still cups. Different sorts of cups are associated with different social contexts.

Now make a list of all features common to your cups.

Ours all held something—even the cup of cheer. If we omitted the cup of cheer image, all our cups were made out of solid enough material to hold something. If we omitted the woman's brassiere and the golf green cups, then we could say they also had handles.

Box 3-1
An Exercise in Creating a Concept and Exploring Various Complex Dimensions of Concepts—cont'd

Let's assume the type of cup you are interested in is a cup for drinking liquid. You now have (1) an object that is made out of solid material that (2) holds something, which means it has an open end and a closed end with (3) a handle.

How do you know this is not a drinking glass that is also used for drinking liquid?

If you said, "It's the handle," you agree with us. We drink liquid from glasses, and they must be made from solid material to hold what we drink. Cups, it seems, need that handle because they usually hold something hot.

Are you getting tired about now? Well, you are in luck because your best friend just came by with some take-out coffee. Out of the bag it comes. Here is a coffee cup without a handle! How can that be?

The technologic development of new materials has omitted the necessity for a handle on cups that hold hot liquids. This tells us that the images associated with cups may change in our lifetime.

Think about the implications of this short mental gymnastic. Cup is a very empiric concept that should be fairly easy to define, yet it isn't. Nursing practice concepts are highly abstract. If cup can get complicated, what challenges will abstract concepts pose when we try to create conceptual meaning?

The point: Conceptual meaning is complex to determine, context determines meaning, and it is critical to know the level of precision needed!

---

validate meanings that are projected by analytic processes. Our approaches to creating conceptual meaning draw on these sources and our experiences of creating conceptual meaning for various purposes.

Selecting a Concept. Selecting a concept is a process that involves a great deal of ambiguity. Concept selection is guided by purpose and always expresses the values of the person who is choosing. If you are a student in a nursing class, your concept selection may be guided by expediency as well as interest. If you are a postdoctoral student, you may be led to create conceptual meaning by a dilemma you encounter in moving through the research process.

Value questions around which concept to select include beliefs, values, and attitudes about the nature of nursing. We believe concepts selected for clarification should justifiably relate to the practice of nursing. An example would be a concept that represents a human response to health or illness, such as fatigue. Characteristics of clients, such as hardiness, may also be selected, particularly if they are important determinants of health. Characteristics of nurses, care systems, or nurse-client-family interaction might also be chosen if they are important determiners of client health. Sociopolitical considerations also influence your choice of a concept, often in ways that are subtle and difficult to perceive. For example, if you choose to examine the concept of transition for daughters who must place their mothers in nursing homes, you will eventually come to examine the consequences of women's caretaking within a society that devalues the elderly.

Some concepts are not appropriate for clarification processes. Some are too empirically grounded, and others are too expansive to yield a useful outcome. Concepts that represent empirically knowable objects (like antiembolic stockings) are usually not good choices because they are highly empirically grounded and can be demonstrated by a display of the thing itself. You do not need concept clarification to understand their meanings, and having criteria for recognizing them will not help you clinically in any significant way. Broad concepts like caring and stress pose another set of problems. Because these types of concepts are so vast, creating meaning can result only in a broad understanding that omits detail and may be misleading. This is not to say that creating conceptual meaning for very narrow or broad concepts is never useful, and some purposes may justifiably require detailed clarification. In our experience, the concepts that work best for clarification processes are those in the midrange. Moreover, it is often helpful when choosing a concept to place it within a context to narrow its scope in relation to your purpose.

Ideally, it makes sense to choose a concept that little is known about as appropriate for creating conceptual meaning. This should not be a primary consideration, however, because the nature of criteria will flex and alter as contexts for use change. Moreover, much of what is in the literature about concepts will be found to be inadequate or erroneous when you examine the concept in the context of multiple data sources. For example, much of the early information on fatigue was generated from research on airplane pilots. This information might initially be assumed appropriate for other people in other circumstances, such as people with cancer who are undergoing chemotherapy. Later, it turned out that the fatigue literature was inadequate to understand cancer fatigue, and nurses began to generate knowledge about this particular type of fatigue. Remember that other disciplines do not have the same perspectives and motives for generating conceptual information as do nurses. Although knowledge of nursing concepts within other disciplines may be useful, these other circumstances need to be carefully examined. Moreover, other disciplines have little interest in nursing concepts and contexts and are likely not to examine them. People in other disciplines are not positioned to have access to data sources about our concepts, and any work they do will probably be inadequate for our purposes. People in other disciplines have no way to appreciate the conceptual meanings of concern to nurses. You can use the information from other disciplines to compare and contrast meanings in a nursing context, but approach meanings derived from other disciplines with some skepticism and examine these meanings carefully.

With these guidelines in mind, you can select a word or phrase that communicates the idea you wish to convey. Despite your best efforts to make the perfect initial choice, it will probably change as you explore various meanings. Trying out alternative words becomes part of the process itself. For example, there is no adequate single term for the idea expressed in the phrase "the use of humans as objects." The term *objectification* is close, but it implies some experiences that do not involve the use of humans. The process of working with various terms related to this idea will help to explore various meanings that are possible. Because experience is not adequately expressed in common language, words may seem quite inadequate at first. You may select a common word for a concept and eventually assign a specific definition to the word to suit your particular purposes; you may borrow a word from another language, combine two or more common words to specify a particular meaning, or make up a phrase or a word. Many significant concepts for nursing have not been named. As nurses engage in processes for creating conceptual meaning, a more adequate language for nursing phenomena will be created. Using clarification processes will help to assure naming that is necessary and valuable for nursing's purposes.

Clarifying Your Purpose. To provide a sense of direction, you must know why you are creating conceptual meaning. One purpose is to set boundaries or limits so you do not become hopelessly lost in the process. For example, your purpose might be to work with the concept "dependence" for a research project. Eventually you need a clear conceptualization of dependence, as well as ideas about how to measure or assess dependence. Another purpose might be to differentiate between two closely related concepts such as sympathy and empathy. In this case, your concern is to create definitions that differentiate, based on thorough familiarity with meanings that are possible.

Another reason for creating conceptual meaning is to examine the ways in which concepts are used in existing writings. The concept of intuition, for example, frequently appears in nursing literature with diverse meanings. The meanings conveyed reflect different assumptions about the phenomenon. As you become aware of these meanings, you can explore the extent to which the meanings are consistent with your own purpose.

Other purposes for creating conceptual meaning include generating research hypotheses, formulating nursing diagnoses, and developing computerized databases for clinical decision making. Creating conceptual meaning is also a valuable process for learning critical thinking (Kramer, 1993). Whatever your purpose, keeping that purpose as clear as possible can provide a sense of direction when you seem to be hopelessly lost.

Sources of Evidence. Once a concept has been selected, the process of creating conceptual meaning proceeds by using multiple sources from which you generate and refine criteria that include indicators for the concept. The sources you choose and the extent to which you use various sources depend on your purposes. Early in the process of gathering evidence for the concept, tentative criteria are proposed, and those criteria are refined in light of additional information provided by continued gathering of evidence. We recommend beginning the process of criteria formulation early on so that useful information is not lost. Which sources of evidence to examine first and the number and types of evidence to gather depend on the purposes of clarification.

Exemplar Case. An exemplar case is a description or depiction of a situation, experience, or event that satisfies the statement: "If this is not *X,* then nothing is." The case can be drawn from nursing practice, literature, art, film, or any other source in which the concept is represented or symbolized. If the case is depicted as an object or in some form of media, many rich aspects of the phenomenon can be conveyed by displaying the media for others to experience. Regardless of format for presentation, the case is selected because it represents the concept to the best of your present understanding. For concrete concepts such as cup, an exemplar case is relatively easy. An ordinary teacup, for example, can be presented for everyone to see and hold. The people who examine the object can then verify, "If this is not a cup, then nothing is." To demonstrate the concept red (a property), a model case is more difficult. You can physically present to the group something that you perceive as red in color and find out if they agree that this is what red is.

When you deal with highly abstract concepts, the task of constructing and selecting exemplar cases is more difficult. Usually, exemplar cases of abstract concepts involve experiences and circumstances that are described in words. Exemplar cases may be created from your own experience, or you may find cases in the literature that have been constructed or described by others. For example, to demonstrate an abstract concept like sorrow, a scenario from a novel or film or a rich description of an experience from your practice can be shared with others, who respond to the scenario as a representation of the phenomenon of sorrow.

If you create your own exemplar case, work with your ideas and revise your description until you are satisfied that the case fully represents your concept. For a concept such as mothering, your exemplar case might describe an event: an infant cries, and an adult picks up the infant. The event is a start, but your observers might object, saying that this description represents only the physical act of picking something up and is not necessarily mothering. Your exemplar case develops until there is enough substance that people respond to the case by forming a mental image of mothering. As you build on the scenario of an adult picking up an infant to represent mothering, you could include various circumstances, behaviors, motives, attitudes, and feelings that surround the act of picking up the infant. You paint a picture or tell a story so that people can confirm that this is indeed mothering. As this and other exemplar cases are created, you can compare various meanings in the experience and define commonalities and differences.

It is often useful to alternatively include and exclude various features of exemplar cases to reflect on how central each feature is to the meaning you are creating. In the exemplar case of mothering, the adult might initially be portrayed as female. Later you might portray a man in the same case. In the absence of any evidence one way or the other, you might tentatively decide that the idea of mothering you are creating will be deliberately limited to instances involving women. Because your decision is tentative, you can change your construction for another purpose or circumstance. You can acknowledge the fact that some men mother, but for your purpose your idea deliberately includes the characteristic of women.

While you are working with exemplar cases, pose the question, What makes this an instance of this concept? The responses to this question form the basis for a tentative list of criteria. In early stages, the criteria may be quite detailed and may be the essential characteristics associated with the concept, given the meanings you deliberately decide to include. The criteria are designed to make it possible to recognize the concept when it occurs and to differentiate this concept from related concepts. For example, in the case of mothering you would want to be able to recognize mothering when it happens and distinguish mothering from such related phenomena as caring, nurturing, or helping.

Impressions about the criteria begin to form as you work with your exemplar case. You begin to form ideas about which features are essential and why, as well as their qualitative features. These ideas become the criteria for the concept. Sometimes exemplar cases are presented after clarification is complete. In these instances the exemplar case is similar to a definitional form for the concept. Here we use exemplar cases as a way to create meaning, not to represent it.

Definitions. One source that provides information about conceptual meaning is definitions and word usages of the concept you are exploring. Existing definitions are often circular and do not give a complete sense of meaning for the concept, but they do help to clarify common usages and ideas associated with the concept. Existing definitions often help to identify core elements about objects, perceptions, or feelings that can be represented by the word. They are also useful to trace the origin of words that give clues to core meaning.

Dictionary definitions provide synonyms and antonyms and convey commonly accepted ways in which words are used. They are not designed to explain the full range of perceptions associated with a word, particularly a word that has a unique use with a discipline or represents a relatively abstract concept.

Existing theories provide a source of definitions that sometimes extend beyond the limits of common linguistic usage. Theoretic definitions and ways concepts are used in the context of the theory convey meanings that pertain to the domain of the discipline from which the theory comes.

The term *mother* as defined in the dictionary, for example, refers to the social and biologic role of parenting and includes a few characteristics of the role, such as authority and affection. In the context of psychologic theories, the meanings conveyed with respect to the values, roles, functions, and characters of people who are mothers are almost endless and include parenting, physical care, guilt, responsibility, power, and powerlessness.

Visual Images. Visual images that already exist, such as photographs, cartoons, calendars, paintings, and drawings, are useful sources for creating conceptual meaning. If you are choosing existing images, they may be explicitly labeled or named as the concept of interest, or you may judge them to reasonably represent it. If you can find images that others have explicitly labeled as an instance of the concept, such as a picture that the artist labels *sorrow,* the artist's link of the visual image and the concept provides further validation of the meaning of the concept, enriches the range of meaning, and helps to minimize any bias inherent in your own views of meaning for the concept.

In some instances you might deliberately create images that represent the concept being clarified rather than use existing sources. Whether you personally create and examine an image or ask others to create images, the idea is to compare them for similarities and differences. Advertisements and photographs documenting the concept depression, for example, provide information about conceptual meaning. Often, visual imagery will highlight some aspect of the concept that is significant. On other occasions, visual imagery may raise questions about the essential nature of the phenomena that are important to refining criteria. Visual images that represent concepts very well also highlight difficulties in expressing meaning linguistically. A photograph may express rich dimensions of the concept of dignity, yet the essence of dignity expressed by the photo is impossible to describe. This is an example of how aesthetic expressions of concepts contribute to empirical knowledge.

Popular and Classical Literature. A variety of literature resources can provide information about conceptual meaning. Literature reflects meanings arising from the culture and provides rich sources of exemplars for concepts. Classical prose and poetry are often rich sources of meaning for concepts used in nursing. For example, images of love and longing may be found in the poetic works of Emily Dickinson. Louisa May Alcott's classic book, *Little Women,* provides information about the nature of intimacy and caring. The popular current literature is also a source of valuable data about conceptual meaning. Popular self-help books on such topics as stress management and codependency can often clarify commonly understood conceptual meanings. Fairy tales, myths, fables, and stories provide relevant insights, depending on the concept you are exploring. Usages for words that are expressed in popular jargon and cartoons may highlight borderline meanings. For example, when a 5-year-old jumps up and down and exclaims, "I'm so anxious for my birthday to be here!" the meaning of *anxious* is not the same meaning that concerns nurses. What the child's usage does convey is the physical agitation that accompanies the experience of anxiety within the context of nursing practice.

Music and Poetry. The imagery of music or poetry may be useful in concept clarification. Music or poetry can be chosen by seeking out lyrics or titles that name the concept under consideration, or the music itself, or the metaphoric images in the title or lyrics, may reasonably suggest the concept. Music and poetry can effectively convey meanings through rhythm, tones, lyrical or linguistic forms and metaphors, or musical moods that reflect experiences in life events with which nurses deal. For example, the Shaker folk tune "Simple Gifts" suggests criteria for concepts of authenticity, genuineness, centeredness, and community. The tune itself conveys a sense of inner happiness and peace; the lyrics reflect relationships between inner peace and the ability to build strong relationships. The popular song "Don't Fence Me In" conveys through the musical mood, rhythm, and lyrics what it feels like to be confined emotionally and projects a yearning to be free.

Professional Literature. Meanings for concepts can be explored from within the context of professional literature. This literature often provides meanings that are pertinent to the practice of nursing. For example, philosophers, as well as nurses, have written about the concept of presence as a way of being with another. Both are valuable sources for exploring meanings. When the literature of other disciplines is considered, meanings may not clearly apply to nursing, but meaning found across disciplines contributes to concept clarification.

People. Peers, co-workers, hospitalized individuals, other professional workers, and people who are not connected to nursing can provide valuable information about the meaning of a concept. It may be useful to seek the others' opinions about the meaning of a concept, particularly if your direct experience with the concept is limited. Nurses who work with the concept daily may be able to shed light on nuances of meaning that will markedly affect how meaning is integrated into theory. For example, a nurse who works with people whose lung function is severely compromised might observe that anxiety, although usually characterized by increased activity, evokes a different reaction. Rather than random activity, anxiety may be accompanied by a deliberate quieting of behavior to conserve energy. Asking others to share their ideas about a concept is an informal exploration different from standard research procedures that might investigate conceptual meaning. Rather, it is an exploration of opinions and understandings of others as a clarification technique.

Methods for Testing Tentative Criteria and the Exemplar Case. As you examine various sources of evidence, you will begin the process of testing the soundness of your conceptualization in light of your purpose. You may find alternate meanings that are plausible but not well suited for your purpose. For example, for someone who is interested in a cup used for the purpose of drinking liquids, a golf green cup, while a plausible instance of the concept of cup, does not have the defining features required for drinking liquids. To stimulate your thinking about nuances of meaning, you can turn to a number of cases that challenge your conceptualization and consider alternate contexts.

Contrary Cases. Contrary cases are those that are certainly not an instance of the concept. They may be similar in some respects, but they represent something that most observers would recognize easily as significantly different from the concept you are considering. For more concrete concepts, contrary cases are relatively easy. A saucer or a spoon can be presented, and most observers in Western cultures would agree that these things are not cups. A spoon may hold liquids that people sip, but it is not a cup. A saucer that a cup sits on is also clearly not a cup. A contrary case for the color red might be the color green. For the concept of restlessness, calmness could be presented as a contrary case.

As you consider contrary cases, ask, What makes this instance different from the concept that was selected? By comparing the differences between exemplar and contrary cases, you will begin to revise, add to, or delete from the tentative list of criteria that are emerging. If your purpose includes designing an exemplar case for your concept, you might also use this information to refine the exemplar case. For example, one of the traits that distinguishes a cup from a saucer or a spoon is the shape of the cup. You might already discern that this feature is essential by looking only at the cup. When you see the spoon and saucer, however, the shape stands out in sharp contrast, and your description of essential features of the shape of the cup can be more complete and precise. As you compare the objects, you may also decide that the volume of liquid that a cup holds is an important distinguishing characteristic. Later, when you consider miniature teacups as cases, you might decide that volume is not an essential quality, especially if your other criteria are sufficient to distinguish which objects can be called a cup for your purpose.

Sometimes in creating narrative contrary cases, the tendency is to simply reverse the situation depicted in the exemplar case. Usually this does not add significant new information to the analysis. If you are having difficulty constructing a negative case, ask someone else to suggest a contrary case or something that is definitely not what you are trying to describe. Sometimes you can locate a contrary case in the literature. Contrary cases that contribute to the analysis often reveal important aspects of the exemplar case that are hidden in assumptions that you may be making about the concept.

Related Cases. Related cases are instances that represent a different but similar concept. Related cases usually share several criteria with the concept being clarified, but one or more criteria will be particularly associated with your selected concept. A different word is generally used to label the related instances. If you find that one word is typically used to refer to essentially different phenomena, you may need to select language for your concept that differentiates it from the related meanings. For example, if you were to be clarifying the concept of love between a parent and child, you may need to use the word label *parental love* to signify that you see essential differences between this experience of love and other related experiences of love.

In the case of a cup, you might consider a drinking glass. For the concept of red, you might consider a red-orange hue and magenta. For the concept of mothering, you could design a case of tending that would be similar to the exemplar case. You might make a child-care worker the adult or substitute an elderly person for the infant. Again you consider differences and similarities between the exemplar and related cases and revise the tentative criteria to reflect your new insights.

Borderline Cases. A borderline case is usually an instance of metaphoric or pseudoapplications of the word. A borderline case is found when the same word is used in a different context. For example, if you are examining fatigue in chronic illness, a useful borderline case of fatigue would be military fatigue clothing. Poetry and lyrics to music provide rich sources of metaphoric uses of words. In the evolution of language the metaphoric meanings of words carry powerful messages that often persist as new usages emerge and thus illuminate core meaning. The metaphoric meanings for the concept of red are excellent examples. *Red* as a word and as a color has become in Western culture a metaphoric symbol for communism, violence, passion, and anger. To give a "cup of cheer" is an exemplary borderline usage of the term *cup*. This highlights the feature of cups as capable of holding something.

For the concept of mothering a borderline case could be a computer motherboard. You might use this borderline usage to help clarify features of the concept of mother that can be seen as foundational to the concept of mothering. These features could include the central importance of mother in defining the scope of relationships or in structuring the energy of all relationships in the system. Ask what happens to your meaning if you perceive mothering as a process that structures and directs the nature of relationships in a system.

Paradoxic cases are variants of borderline cases that are useful to highlight central meanings of concepts. These cases, paradoxically, embody elements of both exemplar and contrary cases. For example, in exploring the meaning of dignity you might create a case in which things that reduce dignity must be done to preserve a central feature of dignity. Such a case is paradoxic in that it violates some criteria for dignity but highlights the importance of a central criterion for discerning the concept.

You will probably invent other varieties of cases in the process of creating conceptual meaning. How cases are classified is not critical. Their important function is to assist you in discerning the full range of possible meaning so that you can design a meaning that is useful for your purpose.

Exploring Contexts and Values. Social contexts within which experience and the values that grow out of experience occur provide important cultural meanings that influence mental representations of that experience. Consider, for example, the concept of judgment if you are a student taking an examination, a Realtor assessing a home for sale, an official scoring a gymnastics meet, or a magistrate preparing to levy a sentence. When you explore the various meanings acquired by virtue of the context, you will probably become aware of meanings you had not previously considered.

One way to imagine various contexts is to place your exemplar cases in different contexts and ask, What next? You mentally imagine the practical outcomes of your conceptual meaning in its context. For example, if you place your exemplar case of the color red in the context of a magazine advertisement, what symbolic meaning is conveyed? What advertising results does the advertiser intend? If the color red is placed in the context of traffic signs and symbols, what meaning does the color now convey? What behavioral responses do you now expect? As you consider various possible combinations of context, you will clarify how meanings are influenced by the context.

Values are also revealed by placing the concept in a subtly differing context. The concept of mothering has a relatively positive connotation for most people. Most people agree that humans need "good" mothering to grow and develop adequately. But people differ widely in what they consider to be good mothering; these differences often have to do with the cultural context. For example, there would probably be considerable disagreement as to whether what happens in a schoolroom, in a hospital, or in counseling is mothering. What is considered mothering reflects deeply embedded cultural values. When you consider your exemplar case placed in several different social contexts, you create an avenue for perceiving important values and make deliberate choices concerning them.

Formulating Criteria for Concepts. We focus on criteria as an expression of conceptual meaning because they are a sensitive and succinct form for conveying essential conceptual meaning that is particularly useful in moving toward other processes of empiric theory development. However, your exemplar case is itself a full expression of conceptual meaning. Other forms of narrative, diagrams, and symbols can express meanings that move beyond the limits of empirics alone. Criteria are necessary and valuable when your purposes include developing formal theoretic structures or research programs to explain empiric phenomena.

Criteria for the concept emerge gradually and continuously as you consider definitions, various cases, other sources, and varying contexts and values. Criteria are always tentative, but they provide guidelines for recognizing the experience you want to represent and for differentiating it from other similar instances.

As you develop the criteria, you will naturally refine them so that they reflect the meaning you intend. Criteria often express both qualitative and quantitative aspects of meaning and should suggest a definition of the word. Because criteria are more complex than a limited word definition, they amplify this meaning and suggest direction for the processes of developing theory.

To illustrate the function of criteria for a concept, consider how you might convey the idea of one U.S. dollar in coins to a person who is not familiar with American money. One way is to present all possible combinations of coins to the individual, who then memorizes the combinations in order to consistently collect the right coins together to yield an equivalent of a dollar. Another approach is to provide guidelines that enable the individual to recognize and compose the various combinations independently. A exemplar case might use three quarters, one dime, two nickels, and five pennies. Because many other combinations are possible, criteria are created from the exemplar case to cover all other possible combinations. The exemplar case is chosen deliberately to include all the types of coins available, so that in examining the case several characteristics of all possibilities emerge. One feature is that the units of the various coins add up to an equivalent of 100 pennies—the smallest possible coin value. However, this criterion alone may not be sufficient for someone who is not familiar with this monetary system, and other criteria are created to ensure that all other possible combinations are recognized. You might consider the weight of the possible coin combinations, the colors of the coins, their metallic makeup, or the exchange value of each coin. All of these features may be used, but criteria should convey, as simply as possible, the information needed by a novice to collect one U.S. dollar in coins. The fact is that any color combination or any number of coins up to 100 may be used as criteria. Metallic content of the coins might serve as an adequate criterion and may even be the most precise of all possible criteria. But if your purpose is to assist a person from another country to understand how to make a dollar's worth of change, you would not select the metallic content as a criterion because it is impractical for that purpose.

For concrete objects criteria may be relatively simple. For the concept of cup examples of criteria may be as follows:

1. The object is cylindric or conic in shape.
2. The object is capable of containing physical matter.
3. The height is between 3 and 7 inches, and the widest diameter is 3 to 4 inches.
4. When the object contains liquid, it must be capable of safely holding hot liquids.

Notice that this set of criteria is phrased so that a Styrofoam cup or golfing green cup can be included. This choice is guided by the purpose. If you needed to make sure that the golfing green cup was not included as a cup, you might revise the criteria to include "the object is capable of being held in the hand, regardless of what it contains." This criterion places a limit on the volume and weight of the cup and implies that it must be a portable object.

Developing criteria for more abstract concepts is a more complex process, and the criteria are often more abstract. Criteria for the concept of mothering might be:

1. Visual contact must be observed to be directed from the mothering person to the person who receives mothering.
2. The person who receives mothering must be physically touched by the mothering person.
3. Some positive feeling must be experienced by the mothering person and by the person who receives mothering.
4. There must be a reciprocal interaction between the mothering person and the person who receives mothering.
5. Vocalization by the mothering person must occur.

These criteria do not limit the mothering person by gender, age, or species. The mother could be an elderly, male person. Nor do the criteria specify that the person who receives mothering is an infant. If the purpose of applying the criteria is to distinguish between instances of mothering and fathering, these criteria would need to be revised to specify at least gender. If the purpose is to differentiate between mothering and neglect, they might be adequate.

A frequent question that arises in the course of creating conceptual meaning is, How do I know that the meaning I have created is adequate? You can examine your conceptual meaning for adequacy in relation to the processes used for creating meaning, as well as the conceptual meaning itself that you have created. Fuller (1991) suggests examining the process and the product of conceptualization in terms of both validity and reliability. A conceptualization is valid if it is based on multiple examples that are fully representative of the range of meanings for the concept, if you used multiple interpretive stages during the clarification process, and if the essential structure (or pattern) of the concept can be understood from the criteria. The conceptualization is reliable if the concept can be consistently recognized on the basis of the criteria that you have created. The meaning you create is also adequate if it reflects a reasonable and communicable understanding that is useful for your purposes. If your aims reflect valued nursing goals, if you have been careful in choosing and using resources, and if you understand why you have made the choices you have, you will have created an adequate and useful meaning. Additional processes for theory development will provide a check on conceptual meaning and will help refine and illuminate whether the meaning created is valuable.

Conceptual Meaning and Problems of Theoretic Development. Problems associated with conceptual meaning often underlie other problems involved in developing theory. A major challenge with respect to generating and testing theoretic relationships is the selection of direct and indirect empiric indicators for a concept. When research reports give conflicting results, the differences are sometimes tied to the use of different definitions and empiric indicators for the concept. If you explore the conceptual meanings within research reports, you can often clarify the extent to which differing conceptual meanings account for the differing research findings. As you carry out the processes for creating conceptual meaning, you will be able to suggest a full range of possible empiric indicators for a concept. You will also be able to identify the limits of empiric approaches in specifying indicators for a phenomenon.

Consider, for example, the concept of mothering and the sample criteria we gave in the previous section. These criteria include characteristics that can be observed empirically. They are reciprocal interaction, visualization, touch, and vocalization. The criterion that states that "some positive feeling must be experienced by the mothering person and by the person who receives mothering" might be one of the most important distinguishing features of your intended meaning for mothering, but it does not easily lend itself to objective observation. It can be assessed indirectly by asking mothers to describe their feelings.

Conceptual meaning is fundamental if you must distinguish one concept from a closely related one. This is often the case when you are forming theoretic relationships or structuring and contextualizing theoretic statements. The processes of creating conceptual meaning make it possible to propose differentiating features that guide research and theory-structuring activities. Consider the concepts of tending and mothering. Individuals tend to the needs of others in many different contexts, and mothers tend children. A question to be resolved might be, is there a particular kind of tending that occurs in mothering? You can examine a related case of a sitter tending children to determine if any characteristic of tending is within your idea of mothering. As you explore various differentiating features of the central concept, your ideas will become clearer, and the structure of your theory or research study will improve. Creating conceptual meaning helps you make decisions about the qualitative dimensions of criteria, such as whether they always need to be evident or if they may be expressed with different intensities. For example, you may decide that, for the concept of mothering, the expression of positive feeling *must* be present, but the degree to which it occurs may vary.

In creating conceptual meaning, the challenge is to evolve a useful and adequate meaning from a range of possibilities. Although the processes for creating conceptual meaning are in and of themselves useful, you move toward refinements of your meaning that are useful for the full range of research, practice, and theory development when you also project how you mean it to be applied in other activities of theory development.

Structuring and Contextualizing Theory

Structuring theory and contextualizing it involve forming systematic linkages between and among concepts, resulting in a formal theoretic structure. Many approaches can be used (Dubin, 1978; Newman, 1979; Reynolds, 1971; Walker and Avant, 1995). The choice of a particular approach depends on your purposes for developing theory, what you already know or assume to be true, and your underlying philosophic ideas about the nature of nursing knowledge. If you begin with an entirely new idea about something and with very little reported about it in the existing literature, the form of the theory that you construct may be a categorization of the concepts into a relational taxonomy that essentially describes your ideas. If you begin with an idea that builds on other theorists' descriptions, you might develop a theoretic structure that provides explanations of complex interrelationships between concepts. If you are structuring theory as an outcome of grounded research, the interrelationships between data clusters guide the structure you create for the theory.

Approaches to structuring and contextualizing theory include the following:

- Identifying and defining the concepts. Identifying and defining concepts specify the ideas on which the theoretic structure is built. Definitions can evolve from the processes of creating conceptual meaning, be borrowed from other theories, or be formulated from multiple other sources. They should identify as clearly and concisely as possible the theoretic meaning of important concepts within the theory.
- Identifying assumptions. Identifying assumptions clarifies the basic underlying truths from which and within which theoretic reasoning proceeds.
- Clarifying the context within which the theory is placed. Contextual placement describes the circumstances within which the theoretic relationships are expected to be empirically relevant. Clear statements regarding context are particularly important if the theory is to be applied in practice.
- Designing relationship statements. Designing theoretic statements describes the projected and evolving relationships between and among the concepts of the theory. These statements, taken as a whole, provide the substance and the form of the theory.

Identifying and Defining Concepts. Structuring theory requires that you identify the concepts that will form the basic fabric of theory. The concepts can come from life experiences, clinical practice, basic or applied research, knowledge of the literature, and the formal processes of creating conceptual meaning. Often theory emerges because of a conviction that existing knowledge and theories are not adequate to represent an experience.

Some concepts are better suited for theory development than others. Concepts that are extremely abstract carry broad meanings and refer to a wide range of experience. They are usually not suitable as a beginning point for theory development. Concepts such as social structure, politics, or love, for example, refer to such a broad range of experience that defining them within the limits of empiric inquiry is extremely difficult. Such concepts, however, can be useful in considering the context within which the theory is placed. If concepts are extremely narrow and concrete, they refer to only a narrow range of experiences, and the level of abstraction may not be sufficient for theoretic purposes. For example, concepts such as toothache, postsurgical pain, or backache apply to relatively few instances of pain. Pain may be a more suitable concept from which to develop theory. What is considered a suitable level of abstraction for theory varies in nursing. The recent trend toward midrange theory provides a useful guideline for decisions about the level of abstraction for theoretic concepts.

As the concepts are specified or begin to form, early ideas about the structure of their relationships begin to emerge. There are usually one or two primary or central concepts around which the theoretic relationships build. Thinking about possible relationships helps to clarify what concepts the theory needs to include. Previous research, existing theories, philosophies, and personal experience provide a background for forming theoretic relationships. Initially, you might simply note concepts that you think are related on the basis of your experience, what you find in the literature, or ongoing research.

An assumption that is inherent in most empiric theory is the concept of linear time. If your emerging theory is to be predictive, time may influence the type and substance of the concepts required for the theory. Antecedent, coincident or intervening, and consequent concepts imply prediction within a linear time frame. Antecedent concepts are those experiences that you identify as coming before other concepts. Coincident concepts are those that coexist in time. Intervening concepts are also coincident and have a particular influence on relationships among concepts that are specified in the theory. Consequent concepts are those that follow another.

Some theories place antecedents in a causal relationship with those that follow. Other theories rest on a philosophic view that rejects the idea of causation. Instead, the ideas of influence or affect are used to explain relationships over time. If a primary concept within your developing theory is stress, you might propose that previous childhood experiences cause the stress experience, or you might consider childhood experience as an antecedent that influences the stress experience.

Consequents can also imply causation. For example, once a person experiences stress, consequents of that experience can be thought of as resulting from the stress. Changes in mental functioning, in sleep and rest patterns, and in relationships with other people might be theoretic concepts structured to reflect phenomena caused by the stress.

Intervening concepts can be used to shift from a view of causation to one of influence. Intervening concepts are those that influence the relationships between antecedent experiences, the event itself, and its consequents. For example, the central concept of stress might be viewed as being influenced by the antecedent experiences of childhood, and sleep patterns might be viewed as an intervening variable that influences the relationship between the childhood experience and present stress.

As initial ideas are formed concerning relationships between concepts, the concepts themselves become clearer, and processes of creating conceptual meaning can be used to make the meanings explicit. Some concepts might be grouped together and assigned more abstract terms to compose a new concept. This occurs especially when theory is structured and conceptualized with inductive theory development processes such as grounded theory. For example, you might begin to see that time of day and season of year could be grouped to become components of the more abstract concept of biologic rhythms.

As the concepts of the theory are identified and conceptualized, theoretic definitions emerge. Theoretic definitions form the basis for and reflect empiric indicators and operational definitions for concepts that are needed for research and convey the general meaning of the concept. Operational definitions are different from theoretic definitions in that they indicate as exactly as possible how the concept is to be assessed in a specific study. For example, a theoretic definition for the concept of mothering might read as follows:

> **mothering** An interaction between a human adult and a child that conveys reciprocal feelings of attachment. The interaction is behaviorally expressed by reciprocal visual contact, touching, and vocalization.

This theoretic definition gives a general idea of the concept's empiric indicators, which in turn imply operational definitions. The first part of the definition provides a general meaning for the term. The second part suggests behaviors associated with the concept that can be assessed.

Notice that the theoretic definition is consistent with tentative criteria for the concept mothering, but the definition serves a different purpose. The criteria are specific and useful as a foundation for construction of theory and for empiric study of the concept. The theoretic definition summarizes the insights that are formed in creating conceptual meaning and concisely conveys the essential meaning of the concept.

Identifying Assumptions as Part of Theory. Assumptions are underlying givens that are presumed to be true. They are not intended to be empirically tested for soundness, but they can be challenged philosophically and may be investigated empirically. Philosophic assumptions form the philosophic grounding for a theory; if they are challenged, the substance of the entire theory is also challenged on philosophic grounds. Nonphilosophic assumptions (that is, assumptions that could be empirically investigated but are not within the context of the theory) also affect the value of the entire theory. Stated assumptions are easy to recognize, but many assumptions are implied or not stated and are difficult to recognize. An example of an underlying assumption that is usually not stated is that human beings are separate from their environment. For theories that involve human experience, this statement can be taken as reasonably true. However, many commonly accepted truths about human existence gain new significance within a theoretic context, and they need to be stated even if they seem self-evident. For example, if a theory includes the concept death, certain underlying assumptions about the nature of life and death would influence the essential ideas of the theory, and these assumptions need to be stated. A theory that is based on a view of death as a transition to another form of life will be very different from a theory that views death as the end of life.

Rogers (1970) made her assumption explicit that human beings are unified wholes, possessing their own integrity and manifesting characteristics that are more than and different from the sum of their parts. On the surface, this statement seems perfectly reasonable and sensible, but it is significant because it is an assumption that is not common to all nursing theory. As an assumption, it does not require empiric evidence, but it is fundamental to the relationship statements Rogers proposed. In theory, it is the relationships, not the assumptions, that are empirically tested.

Assumptions influence all aspects of structuring and contextualizing theory. If the assumption wholism is used as a basis for a theory of mothering, interrelated concepts must be consistent with a holistic view of human experience. Patterns of behavior that reflect the whole would be reflected in the theoretic concepts. They might include patterns of movement and communication. In contrast, if human beings were assumed to be biologic and social organisms, the concepts of a mothering theory might include physical responses and cultural mores.

Clarifying the Context. Theoretic relationships must be placed within a context if the theory is to be useful for practice. If a theory of mothering is meant to apply only to the interactions of women and children in Western cultures, these limits on the applicability of the theory must be stated. As the theory is extended, it might be useful for other cultures and for other kinds of intimate relationships such as adult-child, adult-adult, or adult-animal interactions. Theory that arises from inductive methods is contextualized as a result of the process itself.

Contexts that are very broad or very narrow limit the applicability of theory. A theory that is cognitively structured as an explanation for many cultures will probably not be useful for any culture. Conversely, a theory that is structured within the context of a single institution (for example, one hospital) will probably not be useful for other settings.

Designing Relationship Statements. Relationship statements describe, explain, or predict the nature of the interactions between the concepts of the theory. The statements range from those that simply relate two concepts to relatively complex statements that account for interactions among three or more concepts. Theories usually contain several levels of relationship statements, which comprise a reasonably complete explanation of how the concepts of the theory interact. The relationships begin to take form as the concepts are identified and emerge, but the process of designing the relationship statements requires specific attention to the substance, direction, strength, and quality of interactions between concepts.

Consider a relationship statement that might be formulated about the concept of mothering. A theorist might propose that, as an adult's visual contact with an infant increases, the infant's visual contact with the adult will also increase. This relationship statement speculates that one event (increased adult visual contact) precedes a second event (increased infant visual contact). This relationship also describes a substantive interaction (visual contact) as a component of mothering. It implies direction (an increase) as part of the interaction.

A more complex relational statement addresses further dimensions of quality, contexts, and circumstances that are proposed. Such a statement might take the following form:

Under the conditions of C1 . . . Cn, if X occurs, then Y will occur.

The illustration involving the concept of mothering might take the following form:

When an adult mothering figure and
an infant are in close proximity (C1),
and
when the adult has a negative feeling toward the infant (C2),
and
when the frequency of physical contact is limited (C3),
then,
if the adult's frequency of visual contact decreases,
the infant's frequency of visual contact will also decrease.

A relationship may also be designed to introduce new concepts to the potential theory. Initially, such a relationship might read as follows:

If the infant's frequency of visual contact is not sufficient to satisfy the mother, the adult's frequency of visual contact will increase in a conscious effort to engage the infant in interaction.

This relationship introduces the concept of awareness as well as the subjective value of "sufficient to satisfy." The idea of awareness and a value of sufficiency are not objectively identifiable nor empirically observable. As the theory is developed further, possible empiric indicators for satisfaction might be created, or this dimension of the theory might be viewed as something to be subjectively assessed. In this way the theory not only stimulates the creation of new empiric knowledge but also opens possibilities for exploring and integrating other ways of knowing. Although empiric theory is primarily designed to propose and create empiric relationships, it often contains concepts and relationships that integrate ethical, aesthetic, and personal knowing.

A hypothesis is a type of propositional statement. It is a single statement of a proposed relationship between two or more variables. Hypotheses can take several forms and still provide a basis for developing theory. A neutral hypothesis asserts that one variable *(X)* is related to a second variable *(Y)* or that one variable *(X)* changes in relation to another *(Y)* without indicating the direction of change. A directional hypothesis indicates the direction of association between variables where, as one variable *(X)* increases or decreases, a second *(Y)* also increases or decreases.

A confirmed hypothesis is a relationship statement for which there is research support. It can be either directional or neutral. Hypothesis testing requires that certain controls and procedures be adhered to and that statistical exemplars be applied in the confirmation process.

The traditional form of expressing hypotheses requires statements that conform to rules of logic. The logic may be either deductive or inductive. The following sections provide an overview of each of these forms of logic. Box 3-2 explains deductive and inductive forms of logic that are often used or that provide a foundation for constructing formal hypotheses.

Comparison of Induction and Deduction. Deductive logic is reasoning from the general to the particular. Inductive logic is reasoning from the particular to the general. In inductive logic particular instances are observed to be consistently part of a larger whole or set, and the set of particular instances is merged with that larger whole. This larger set can then be considered in relation to still another set of events or phenomena in another logical system.

In deductive logic the premises as starting points embody two variables that can be categorized in relation to each other as broad or specific. In Box 3-2 humans (a broad concept) were said to use cups with handles (a specific feature). In the other premise, neonates were said to be a class of humans: that is, neonates were specifically members of a broader class (humans). The

Box 3-2
Understanding Logic as a Formal System of Reasoning

DEDUCTION

FORMAT	EXAMPLE A	EXAMPLE B
A is B (premise)	The "fit" survive	Humans use cups with handles
C is A (premise)	The most numerous are the "fit"	Neonates are humans
C is B (conclusion)	The most numerous survive	Neonates use cups with handles

What to Know:

- Sound conclusions can be empirically empty, as in example A, where both premises are definitionally true but give no new information.
- Conclusions are only as sound as premises, as in example B, where the format is correct but the first premise is not true.
- Premises go by several labels: hypotheses, suppositions, axioms, or propositions.
- Conclusions go by several labels: laws or theorems.
- Reasoning moves from general to particular: the conclusion is a specific instance of first premise
- Deduction is associated with the hypotheticodeductive methodology of traditional science.
- Challenge: to use premises that have enough empiric confirmation to yield useful theoretic constructions.

INDUCTION

FORMAT	EXAMPLE A	EXAMPLE B
X_1 is a member of set Y associated with Z.	A grackle is a black bird and can fly.	A bunionectomy is a painful surgical procedure.
X_2 is a member of set Y associated with Z.	A starling is a black bird and can fly.	A laparotomy is a painful surgical procedure.
X_3 is a member of set Y associated with Z	A crow is a black bird and can fly.	A tooth extraction is a painful surgical procedure.
X_4 is a member of set Y associated with Z.	A raven is a black bird and can fly.	A closed reduction is a painful surgical procedure.
X_5 is a member of set Y associated with Z.	A vulture is a black bird and can fly.	A tendon repair is a painful surgical procedure.
Therefore, $X_6, X_7 \ldots X_n$ are members of set Y and associated with Z.	Therefore, All black birds can fly.	Therefore, All surgical procedures are painful.

Box 3-2

Understanding Logic as a Formal
System of Reasoning—cont'd

What to Know

- The observation of multiple particular instances of the same phenomena that share a common characteristic is required to generalize that all subsequent cases will also share that characteristic.
- Reasons from the particular to the general case.
- Induction is associated with the inductive research methodologies.
- Challenge: to observe enough instances of individual instances to have confidence in the generalization.

---

conclusion contains both specific variables: neonates use cups with handles. In deductive logic, the movement is from premises embodying broad and specific variables to a conclusion in which the variables are more specific.

Like most other words, *deduction* and *induction* have common meanings related to, but different from, their meaning within systems of logic. People often state that they deduce hypotheses from theory or deductively develop theory. These deductions are not the result of applying rules of logic but arise out of careful thought without specifically using a system of logic. Used like this, deduction implies that a more general theory was a source of specific hypotheses or relational statements.

With induction, people induce hypotheses and relationships by observing or experiencing an empiric reality and reaching some conclusion. These related meanings of induction and deduction should be noted because sometimes the terms refer to systems of logic and to rules and conventions for the ordering of reasoning. At other times the terms refer to a general approach to thinking, short of logical rules but similar in form.

CONCLUSION

The interrelated processes for theory development include creating conceptual meaning and structuring and contextualizing theory. Although theory, as we have defined it, can be developed by using only conceptual approaches, for theory to be useful in practice, research will be an integral part of the development process. Once a theory has been developed, members of the discipline begin to assess the adequacy of the theory by using methods of creating conceptual meaning, conducting additional research based on the theory, and exploring its applicability in practice. In Chapter 4 we describe methods for assessing the adequacy of theory. Chapter 5 describes research approaches that test a theory's adequacy, and Chapter 6 presents approaches to applying theory deliberatively in practice.

Reference List

Dickoff J, James P: A theory of theories: a position paper, *Nurs Res* 17:197, 1968.

Dubin R: *Theory building* (rev ed), New York, 1978, Free Press.

Ellis R: Characteristics of significant theories, *Nurs Res* 17:217, 1968.

Fuller J: *A conceptualization of presence as a nursing phenomenon.* Unpublished doctoral dissertation, University of Utah, Salt Lake City, UT.

Jacox A: Theory construction in nursing: an overview, *Nurs Res* 23:4, 1974.

Kaplan A: *The conduct of inquiry,* New York, 1964, Thomas Y Crowell.

Kramer M: Concept clarification and critical thinking: integrated processes, *J Nurs Educ* 32:1, 1993.

Levine ME: The four conservation principles of nursing, *Nurs Forum* 6:93, 1967.

McKay RP: Theories, models and systems for nursing, *Nurs Res* 18:393, 1969.

Morse JM: Exploring the theoretical basis of nursing using advanced techniques of concept analysis, *Adv Nurs Sci* 17:31, 1995.

Müller ME, Dzurec LC: The power of the name, *Adv Nurs Sci* 15:15, 1993.

Newman MA: *Theory development in nursing,* Philadelphia, 1979, FA Davis.

Norris CM: *Concept clarification in nursing,* Rockville, Md, 1982, Aspen.

Reynolds PD: *A primer in theory construction,* Indianapolis, 1971, Bobbs-Merrill.

Rogers ME: *An introduction to the theoretical basis of nursing,* Philadelphia, 1970, FA Davis.

Walker LO, Avant KC: *Strategies for theory construction in nursing* (ed 3), Norwalk, Conn, 1995, Appleton & Lange.

Watson J: *Nursing: human science and human care: a theory of nursing,* Norwalk, Conn, 1985, Appleton-Century-Crofts.

Wilson J: *Thinking with concepts,* London, 1963, Cambridge University Press.

Wright MR: Research and research, *Nurs Res* 15:244, 1966.

Chapter 4

Description and Critical Reflection of Empiric Theory

We converse with one another of knowledge, research, assumptions
and so forth, overconfident that we understand.

Norma Koltoff (1967, p. 122)

O nce theories and models are developed, the questions "What is this?"
and "How does it work?" can be asked by anyone with an interest in
using or understanding the theory. This chapter sets forth analytic thought
processes that are useful in understanding the nature and value of theory and
other forms of empiric knowledge, including models and descriptions. These
processes describe theory and critically reflect theory—that is, examine its
value for various purposes. A clear understanding of the nature of theory,
which flows from description and critical reflection, may be undertaken
before engaging in research processes incorporating the theory or attempting to utilize the theory in practice. The questions "What is it?" and "How
does it work?" both stimulate development of theory and serve as an
organizing framework for deliberately examining it.

The definition of theory we use in this text suggests that theory is
comprised of elements that can form the basis for a descriptive scheme.

theory: A creative and rigorous structuring of ideas that projects a tentative,
purposeful, and systematic view of phenomena.

The descriptive components that this definition suggests are as follows:

- *Purpose.* If theory projects a tentative, purposeful, and systematic view of phenomena, it follows that theory and models are developed for some reason that can be identified. The purpose of a theory may not be stated explicitly, but it should be identifiable.
- *Concepts.* If theory represents a structuring of ideas, the ideas will be in the form of concepts that are expressed in language.
- *Definitions.* If theory is intelligible or understandable, which systematization of concepts implies, the concepts of a theory must carry identifiable meanings that are conveyed in definitions. Definitions vary in precision and completeness, but conceptual meaning should be identifiable in a theory. The meanings for the concepts created by the theorist give the theory its particular character.
- *Relationships and structure:* If the concepts are related and structured into a systematic whole, then the overall whole of the theory is identifiable.
- *Assumptions:* If theory is tentative, assumptions form the underlying "taken for granted" truths of the theory's creator and leave open possible theoretic interpretations that would come from different sets of assumptions.

Theory, by definition, contains these identifiable components. Describing theory is a process of posing questions about these components and responding to the questions with your own reading or interpretation of the theory. Some elements will seem clear; some will depend on tentative interpretations; some will remain unclear. Despite ambiguities, the process of describing theory creates an objective description that can then form the basis for critical reflection.

WHAT IS THIS? THE DESCRIPTION OF THE THEORY

In this section we discuss the processes for describing theory. Once a theory is described, the description can be used as a basis for critical reflection. Critical reflection processes follow the description section.

What Is the Purpose of This Theory?

The general purpose of the theory is important because it specifies the context and situations in which the theory applies. Purpose can be initially approached by asking, Why is this theory formulated? Information about the theorist's sociopolitical context provides insight about circumstances that influenced the creation of the theory. The theorist's experience, the setting in which the theory was formulated, societal trends, philosophic ideas that gave form to the theorist's view, and experience that motivated the creation of the ideas of the theory can all provide insight as to why it was formulated. The responses to this question provide information that pertains to theoretic purposes.

For the question of purpose, it is important to clarify which purposes are embedded in the theoretic structure and which are reasonable extensions of the theory. For example, consider a theory of mother-infant attachment that includes the following concepts: (1) birth or adoption experience, (2) maternal support systems, (3) degree of bonding, and (4) healthy infant development. Healthy infant development is an example of a clinical outcome—or purpose—that is embedded in the structure of the theory. Quality of life as a purpose would be an extension of the theory because this concept is not found within the structure of the theory. Purposes that are identifiable within the structure of the theory are usually explicit. Purposes that are reasonable extensions of the theory are important for clarifying the clinical usefulness of the theory, but they are not clearly linked to the central structure of the theory. Purposes outside the context of the theory also suggest directions for further development of the theory.

Some purposes require the practice of nursing to be achieved. In these theories the concepts of the theory include nursing actions and behaviors that contribute to the purpose. Pain alleviation and restored self-care ability are examples of purpose that require the practice of nursing and suggest that nursing actions are part of the theory. Note that these purpose statements have a value orientation: alleviation and restoration. These ideas imply change toward a certain goal, not just change for the sake of change. Value connotations such as these are important to understanding the purpose of the theory.

Some purposes may not require the practice of nursing but are useful for understanding phenomena that occur in the context of nursing practice. These purposes can contribute to achieving practice purposes, or they may not be directly relevant to practice goals. Consider, for example, a theory with a central purpose of explaining variables affecting blood flow velocity in the skin. Clinical practice is not necessary to explain blood flow velocity, but a theory with this purpose might be linked to a theoretic explanation of how blood flow velocity influences the incidence of decubitus or the extent of peripheral neuropathy in people with diabetes. A theory that explains skin blood flow velocity would also help practitioners prevent decubitus and peripheral neuropathy.

Theoretic purposes that do not require direct clinical nursing actions but are of concern to nursing may also involve professional issues in nursing. For example, the purpose of a theory might be to describe features of organizations that empower nurses. This valued and necessary purpose is not directly related to the specific nursing actions of giving care, but it is certainly useful for changing practice.

Purposes within a theory may be found for individuals or for groups of people. For example, if a theory is developed toward the clinical goal of pain alleviation, the theory can be examined for purposes appropriate for the nurse, the physicians, the person receiving care, and the family. Consider theory developed with a clinical purpose of promoting high-level wellness. The role and outcomes for the nurse might be distinctly different from that implied for the person receiving nursing care. The nurse's purpose might be to design a system that promotes recovery. The purpose for the person receiving care might be to recover and to provide responses that indicate how effective the system is in promoting recovery. Taken together, these two purposes might be viewed as creating an interacting recovery process.

One question that often arises is, How are purposes to be separated from the concepts of the theory? Purposes that are part of the matrix of the theory are also concepts of the theory. One approach to identifying which concept is also the central purpose is to describe or to designate the concept toward which theoretic reasoning flows. This is related to the structure of the theory. Ask, What is the end point of this theory? and When is this theory no longer applicable? Responses to these questions provide clues to purpose and help to clarify the context in which the theory can be used. In Hall's (1966) theory, for example, the theory would cease to be valuable when the client was self-actualized, and self-actualization may be deemed the overall purpose. This purpose of self-actualization represents the end point of theoretic reasoning. In the context of Hall's theory self-actualization is a purpose that requires nursing actions. Outside the context of Hall's theory self-actualization is a purpose that is shared with other professions. Hall's theory provides a nursing context within which self-actualization becomes meaningful.

Another question about purpose concerns the individual, family, group, and societal dimensions of the theory. Does the purpose of a theory apply to society? To groups? To individuals? An adapted society and an expanded collective consciousness are examples of broad purposes that apply to relatively unbounded groups of people. Purposes such as environmental health or political activism apply to communities that can be linked to a definable group of people. The purpose of quality of life can apply to individuals, families, groups, and communities.

The scope of a theory refers to the breadth or range of phenomena to which the theory applies. It is often reflected in the theory's purpose. The level of abstraction of the theory's concepts is integral to its scope. Theory may be characterized as micro, macro, molecular, midrange, molar, atomistic, and wholistic. Another term also found in the literature is *grand theory*, meaning theory that covers broad areas of concern within a discipline. *Metatheory* is a term used to designate theory about theory and the processes for developing theory.

Categorizations of scope are relative, and labels that are typically used to classify the scope of theory reflect a continuum of breadth. Micro, molecular, and atomistic, for example, suggest relatively narrow-range phenomena, whereas macro and molar imply that the theory covers a relatively broader range of phenomena. These categories are often relative to the scope of the discipline. What is micro for one discipline may be midrange in others. A theory of wholistic humans would likely be broad in scope in almost any discipline and would deal with patterns reflecting the whole. Grand theory, unlike macro and molar theory, refers to very broad-scope theory in most disciplines. The term *atomistic* implies a narrow scope and has the connotation of assuming that parts are a legitimate focus for study in order to generalize about the whole. Conversely, *wholistic* connotes that the sum of parts cannot reflect the whole.

Micro or molecular theory may reflect purposes that can be known only indirectly because evidence to validate their achievement requires perceptions keener than those provided by unaided senses. The purpose of altering action potential is representative of this category. Improving regional blood flow is an even broader purpose than altering action potential because in some cases it is indirectly perceptible, whereas action potentials cannot be assessed without sensitive signal-processing equipment. Concepts contained in such theories are narrow and often specifically defined.

When the purpose increases in scope to represent a portion of an accepted overall purpose for a profession or discipline, midrange theory is being approached. A theory of pain alleviation is an example of this range because pain alleviation is one of several areas of concern to nursing. Micro theories might attempt to explain the physiology of pain phenomena, whereas midrange theories would deal with pain alleviation as a segment of nursing's total interest. Concepts contained in midrange theory reflect this part of whole orientation; they are broader than those contained in micro theories but still do not reflect the totality of nursing's concern.

Macro theories conceptualize purpose broadly. Health, expanded consciousness, and high-level wellness, not just for individuals but for people in general, are examples of such purposes. Macro theories deal with the whole of nursing's concern. Concepts within these theories tend to be broad in scope and related to individuals as wholes rather than as portions of the person's structure or function.

An example may serve to illustrate how the purpose provides information that can be used in responding to questions about scope. Abdellah and her colleagues (1960) have proposed that nursing purposes can be described as the solution of problems in 21 different categories. Each problem is complex in itself, and taken together they are represented as the totality of nursing function. Problem 11 is "to facilitate maintenance of sensory function." Theory regarding the solution and prevention of sensory function as a problem could be considered midrange theory in that it is only 1 of 21 problems of concern to nursing. Narrower theory is possible concerning the development or maintenance of sensory function in diverse groups, such as those with chronic illness, the young or aged, or any of numerous subdivisions. Theory of sensory neural transport would represent micro theory in relation to this problem area. Assume that the maintenance of function in all 21 problem areas constitutes health, whereas the solution of existing problems constitutes movement from illness toward health, with health a valued purpose for individuals. Macro theory would be theory that interrelates all 21 problem areas so that the general purpose of health restoration or maintenance could be approached.

What Are the Concepts of This Theory?

Concepts are identified by searching out words or groups of words that represent objects, properties, or events within the theory. You can begin to describe concepts by listing key ideas and tentatively identifying how they seem to interrelate. As you begin to discern relationships, your perception of the key concepts of the theory will become clearer. One initial difficulty in identifying concepts is determining which concepts are integral to the theory and which are part of some supporting narrative. There is no easy way to deal with this difficulty. By beginning to identify concepts and deriving interrelationships, decisions can be made about which concepts are central to the theory.

As you identify important theoretic concepts, ask questions about the nature of the concepts and their organization. Is there a major concept with subconcepts organized under it? Are there several major concepts with subconcepts organized under them? Are concepts singular entities? Are some concepts singular entities and others organized with subconcepts? What are the relationships and interrelationships between and among concepts? Are some concepts mentioned that do not seem to fit the emerging structure? What is the relative scope of the various concepts? Once concepts are identified and questions such as these are addressed, the relationships and structure will begin to emerge.

Other questions deal with the numbers of concepts. How many concepts are there? How many might be termed major concepts? How many are minor concepts? Do not get into a conundrum in trying to distinguish between major and minor. Rather, notice whether some one concept or a few concepts really stand out as important while others seem less so, and why. As you consider the organization and quantity of concepts, address qualitative features of the concepts as well. Do the concepts represent abstractions of objects, properties, or events? Is it possible to identify what they represent? Are the concepts more empirically grounded, or are they more abstract? What proportion of the concepts is empirically grounded? What proportion is highly abstract? Are the concepts fairly discrete in meaning, or do several have similar meanings? When similar meanings for concepts exist, do they all seem to express a single idea, or are they different? How? Concepts that are alike may represent one central idea that is fairly clear or several different images. For example, the concepts of rehabilitation, restoration, and recovery, which share common meanings, may appear in the same theory with similar meanings or with different meanings.

When you are addressing the question of a theory's concepts, the concepts within it must be examined carefully for quantity, character, emerging relationships, and structure. The description of concepts is crucial because their quantity and character form understanding of the purpose of the theory, the structure and nature of theoretic relationships, the definitions, and the assumptions.

What Are the Definitions in This Theory?

A definition is any explicit or implicit meaning that is conveyed for a concept. Definitions exist to clarify the nature of the abstraction that the theorist constructs in a way that others can comprehend. Definitions suggest how word representations of an idea (concept) are expressed in empiric reality.

It is often difficult to determine from a listing of key words which concepts are basic to the theoretic structure and which comprise definitions and assumptions. Carefully reading the theory and relying on your own judgment should provide this information.

Concepts may be defined explicitly, such as in a list of definitions, or they may be explicitly defined in narrative form in the text but not labeled as definitions. It is not always easy to recognize implicit definitions because they are not labeled and are often inferred from implied meanings.

Because concepts may be defined both explicitly and implicitly, ask the following questions: How are concepts defined? Explicitly? Implicitly? Both?

Are implied definitions consistent with explicit definitions? Can common language meanings be taken as the meaning intended? Would a common language approach lead to differing interpretations of the meanings of the concepts?

Another way to describe definitions is to characterize the extent to which the definitions are general or specific. It is possible for both explicit and implicit meanings to be either general or specific. Assess how general or specific definitions are. How clearly does the definition suggest an associated empiric experience? Is the definition specific about what a phenomenon is, or does it suggest what it is used for? Does it provide possibilities for empiric indicators that represent the phenomenon?

For abstract concepts found in many nursing theories, specific definitions are difficult to formulate. Attempting to create specific meanings of abstract concepts prematurely may interfere with exploring a wide range of possibilities that lead to discovery. Definitions that specify general features can conjure very specific mental images of the actual experience. An early definition that is broad and nonspecific encourages the exploration of many possible meanings. General meanings are preferred in broad-scope theory or theory that is not likely to be empirically tested. Most definitions have both specific and general features. How are definitions both specific and general?

Once definitions are identified, ask the following questions: Are similar definitions used for different concepts? Are differing definitions used for the same concept? Are some concepts defined differently than common convention? Are definitions expanded as the narrative proceeds? Is it difficult to judge whether definitions are provided at all? Can definitions fit other terms within or outside the structure of the theory?

What Relationships Are in This Theory?

Relationships provide links among and between concepts. The nature of relationships in theory may take several forms. Often relationship statements that are uncovered may be peripheral to the core of the theory.

As concepts are identified, ideas about relationships between them begin to form. Suppose you uncover a relationship statement: "The individual is composed of three dimensions and is an integral part of the environment." This statement suggests that the individual is related to an environment and that there are three interrelated subcomponents of the individual.

Once a tentative identification of relationships is made, ask the following questions: Are there concepts that stand alone, unrelated to others? Are there concepts interrelated with other concepts in several ways and others related in only one or two ways? Are there concepts to which several other concepts relate but that, in turn, are not related to other concepts?

The ways in which the relationships emerge provide clues to the theoretic purposes and the assumptions on which the theory is based. Some concepts may be linked to the theory by assumptions, which may explain why the concept seems to fit within the matrix of the theory but a theoretic relationship containing the concept is not explicitly stated. The theoretic purpose can be represented by the one-way relationships of several concepts with one specific concept that in turn is not linked to any other concepts—that is, the links end with this specific concept. As linkages between concepts are identified, you can address the nature or character of relationships. If a relationship is unclear, ask yourself what relationships might be possible and their character; your ideas can provide clues for further development of the theory.

Examine the nature of the relationships. Are the relationships basically descriptive, or do they explain? Do they create meaning without explaining? Do they impart understanding? Is there evidence that some relationships are predictive? Relationships within theory that create meaning and impart understanding often link multiple concepts in a loose structure. In other forms of description, concepts are interrelated without elaboration on how and why conceptual relationships are arranged. Concepts that are interrelated to explain often convey how empiric events occur and may provide some detail about how and why concepts interrelate. Prediction implies if-then statements about the occurrence of empiric phenomena. When predictions of human behavior are shown to be valid, they are usually based on explanation.

The statement "Individuals are composed of three dimensions" is mainly descriptive. It implies that one concept, the individual, is composed of three parts called dimensions. If expanded to "The individual is composed of three dimensions that overlap and share common core areas," the statement becomes more explanatory. It proposes that each dimension has a shared area with another dimension and that there is an area shared by all three. When "interrelated whole" is added, the "how" of the relationship becomes even clearer because the dimensions must overlap to interrelate the parts of the individual.

Predictions are fairly easy to detect. Sentences that translate into if-then statements are predictive. It is not possible to make an if-then statement out of "The individual is composed of three dimensions," unless it is the implied "If not three dimensions, then not the individual." The statement "The individual is an interrelated whole composed of three dimensions that overlap and share common areas" implies that disturbances in one sphere would be reflected in other spheres. This prediction, however, is not explicit.

Suppose the statement read, "Because the individual is an interrelated whole composed of three dimensions that overlap and share common areas, a disturbance in one dimension is reflected in disturbances in other dimensions." This statement is clearly predictive. The distinctions between description, explanation, and prediction are not always clear. Generally description means that the statement projects what something is or the features of its character. Explanation suggests how or why it is. Prediction projects circumstances that create or alter a phenomenon. Our use of the terms *descriptive, explanatory,* and *predictive* in describing the nature of theoretic relationships refers only to the form of the theory. In this context, we do not mean to imply that empiric validation or findings are required to discern whether relationship statements are descriptive, explanatory, or predictive.

What Is the Structure of This Theory?

The structure of theory gives overall form to the conceptual relationships within it. The structure emerges from the relationships of the theory. Consider two concepts within a theory: individual and environment. In one theory individuals are part of the environment; in another theory individuals are separate from the environment. In both theories there is an identifiable relationship between individuals and environment, but the structure of the relationship differs. Figure 4-1 illustrates a number of possible structural relationships that can be discerned.

Although your responses to questions concerning the relationships of theory usually suggest the form, in some cases they do not. Many theories do not contain a single discernible structure in which all concepts fit into a coherent, unified network. There may be several, perhaps competing, structures that cannot be reconciled. Determining the structure of theory will be difficult if the network of relationships is unclear or very complex. Figure 4-1 depicts a sample of four structural forms and the ideas they suggest. Some theories may reflect one or more of these structures, whereas others will not. Sometimes individual concepts within theories may be structured in these forms. Structural forms are powerful devices for shaping our perceptions of reality. As you describe theory, do not expect that it will fit into one of these four structures. It may, but many more are possible. Conversely, in the process of theory development these are only examples of various structures that might evolve in the process of relationship structuring.

Consider how you might structure the relationship statement "Individuals are composed of component parts." This statement only suggests a structure in which parts are perceptible, and any image on Figure 4-1 could represent it except the one that suggests polarity. Suppose each of these

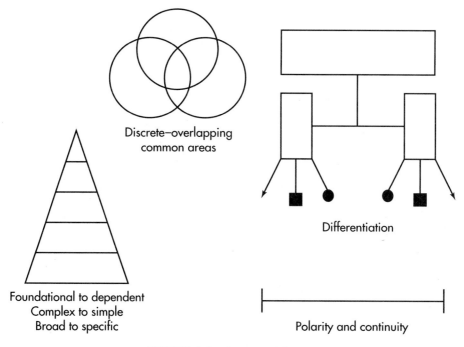

Discrete–overlapping
common areas

Differentiation

Foundational to dependent
Complex to simple
Broad to specific

Polarity and continuity

FIGURE 4-1 Structural forms.

structures represents the broad theory of health. The triangular drawing suggests that health is composed of a series of related subconcepts that vary in breadth or simplicity. It also suggests foundational concepts on which other subconcepts are built. The base level might be genetic integrity, followed by organ-system health, and finally health of communities or societies. A theory that deals with how genetic health forms the basis for individual, collective, and societal health might be structured this way.

The overlapping circles depict discrete components that have common areas between and among them. Health might be viewed as having biophysiologic, psychoemotional, and sociocultural aspects. If a person is biologically well but psychoemotionally unwell, the diagram suggests that illness will affect biophysiologic wellness. Psychoemotional ill health could result in biophysiologic consequences. Basically the overlapping circles illustrate that health is composed of separate components, but there is sharing between any two components, as well as among all three. The structure as illustrated suggests an equality in importance, overlap, and sharing among the three subunits.

Applying this idea to the horizontal line drawing on the figure shows health represented as a continuum—in a linear relationship with illness.

When health is placed on a continuum with illness on the opposite end, health and illness are conceptualized as a continuous variable, and degrees of health and illness are possible. The extremes of a continuum also suggest that health is the absence of illness, and illness is the absence of health. If health is viewed as a concept that is continuous with illness, health and illness can be represented by a continuum. If health and illness are considered as noncontinuous concepts, they do not fit this structural form. A relationship between gender and society could not be represented on a continuum, for example.

The fourth structural form conveys the idea of differentiation, dividing major concepts into subconcepts. For this structural form, health might be differentiated into its mental and physical aspects. Physical health could be further divided into bodily or anatomic health and functional or physiologic health, with some comparable division such as emotional and spiritual for mental health. Differentiation can proceed indefinitely. Some concepts lend themselves to differentiation more easily than others. Needs is a concept that can be easily differentiated, whereas the concept of wholism cannot.

As you study the examples of structure, note how different concepts fit some structures more easily than others and how some concepts such as wholistic health cannot be represented well by any of them. In fact, none of these structures for representing health may make sense for you because they are inconsistent with your personal ideas about the nature of health.

As relationships are explored, the overall theoretic structure and the structures of individual components begin to emerge. To address questions of structure, begin by asking, What are the most central relationships? What are the direction, strength, and quality of relationships? Can I draw a model that shows the structure of the theory? What is the order of appearance of relationships within the narrative? Do relationships appear to move toward or away from the theoretic purpose? Do relationships coalesce concepts or differentiate them? Does the theorist diagram the structure?

Once the structure of the major or central relationships is identified, other aspects of structure can be described. How are other structures united with central or core relationships? Can all relationships be structured? Do the structures take multiple forms? Are competing or partial structures suggested? Does the theorist provide diagrams that illustrate aspects of structure?

Once you have structured the relationships, describe the entire structural form. Notice how the relationships move as the theory unfolds. A theory that defies structuring can sometimes be approached by simply outlining the order in which concepts are presented. Outlining can provide insight about how ideas are organized. Some recognizable structure is essential to theory because structure flows from relationships.

What Assumptions Are in This Theory?

Assumptions are those basic givens or accepted truths that are fundamental to theoretic reasoning. To uncover assumptions, a central question is, What is the author taking as an accepted truth? This question can be asked once the purposes are determined, the concepts are structured by relational statements, and the definitions are described.

Sometimes the theorist states assumptions explicitly. If so, ask, What are they? What do they assume? Statements explicitly labeled assumptions may not be the same as the assumptions that are basic to the theory. The extent to which explicitly labeled assumptions are assumptions and not something else must be examined. It is often difficult to separate assumptions that are implicit or integrated into the narrative of the theory from relationship statements, but they can be identified. As with explicit assumptions, ask, What are the implicit givens? What do they assume?

Explore your ideas about the assumptions of the theory further. What individual, environmental, nursing, and health-related assumptions are made? Are assumptions competing or compatible? Are there several assumptions about one phenomenon and few about another? Are assumptions made at the outset, between and within relationships, or in relation to the purposes of the theory?

Assumptions may take the form of factual assertions, or they may reflect value positions. Factual assumptions are those knowable or potentially knowable through experience. Value assumptions assert or imply what is right, good, or ought to be. Often an empirically knowable assumption such as "It is assumed for the purposes of this theory that people want information" contains important underlying value assumptions. The assumption that people want information (which could be empirically verified) may further imply that information is good, which cannot be verified empirically. The value assumption that it is good to have information leads to further questions about what sort of information is good. It is important to examine factual assumptions by asking, What value does this factual assumption reflect? It is also important to examine all other components of theory. What does this concept, definition, relationship, structure, or purpose assume?

Once you discern assumptions, the values held by the theorist can be explored. What does the theorist assume to be valuable, good, right, wrong, or worthwhile? Are there value-laden terms and phrases in the definitions of concepts and in the supporting narrative of the theory? Who is assumed to be responsible for the experiences or circumstances of the theoretic reality? Who benefits from the circumstances or experiences of this theory? These questions often give clues to values that form fundamental assumptions. For example, the Freudian theoretic notion of penis envy implies that penises are body parts that are so valued as to be enviable and that a person who does not have a penis will experience this value-laden emotion. A useful approach to uncovering hidden values is to imagine possibilities other than that presented in the theory. If these alternate possibilities are plausible but unconventional, you have uncovered important value assumptions. Imagining the idea of womb envy, which is not a part of Freudian thinking but is a plausible alternate possibility, indicates that you have uncovered an important androcentric assumption from which the theory builds.

The descriptive component of assumptions is often based on ideas taken so much for granted that they are difficult to recognize. An example of such an obvious assumption is that reality is what can be perceived and experienced through the senses. This assumption is fundamental to empirics, but it is not an assumption of other patterns of knowing.

Sometimes it is not possible to accept a theory because it is unusual or unfamiliar. Uneasiness or discomfort with a theory is sometimes a clue to assumptions that are unlike your own beliefs or values. Once assumptions are recognized, the theory containing them can be understood on its own terms.

Forming a Complete Description

In summary, the six questions we propose for describing theory are as follows:

1. What is the purpose of this theory? This question addresses why the theory was formulated and reflects the contexts and situations to which the theory can be applied.
2. What are the concepts of this theory? This question identifies the ideas that are structured and related within the theory. It questions the qualitative and quantitative dimensions of concepts.
3. How are the concepts defined? This question clarifies the meaning for concepts within the theory. It questions how empiric experience is represented by the ideas within the theory.
4. What is the nature of relationships? This question addresses how concepts are linked together. It focuses on the various forms relationship statements can take and how they give structure to the theory.
5. What is the structure of the theory? This question addresses the overall form of the conceptual interrelationships. It discerns whether the theory contains partial structures or has one basic form.
6. On what assumptions does the theory build? This question addresses the basic truths that underlie theoretic reasoning. It questions whether assumptions reflect philosophic values or factual assertions.

A general approach to describing theory is to read the work and then begin to consider the descriptive questions. The outline shown in Box 4-1

Box 4-1
Guide for the Description of Theory

1. PURPOSE
- Why is this theory formulated?
- Is there an overall purpose for the theory? A hierarchy of purposes? Separate numerous purposes?
- Is there a purpose for the nurse? The person receiving care? Society? Environment?
- How broad or narrow is the purpose?
- What is the value orientation of the purpose? Positive, negative, neutral?
- Does achieving the theoretic purpose require a nursing context?
- Does [do] the purpose[s] reflect understanding? Creation of meaning? Description, explanation, and prediction of phenomena?
- When would the theory cease to be applicable? What is the end point?
- What purpose not explicitly embedded in the matrix of the theory can be identified?

2. CONCEPTS
- Is there one major concept with subconcepts organized under it?
- How many concepts are there?
- How many major ones?
- How many minor ones?
- Can the concepts be ordered, related? Arranged into any configuration?
- Are there concepts that cannot be interrelated?
- Are concepts broad in scope? Narrow?
- How abstract or empiric are the concepts?
- What is the balance between highly abstract and highly empiric concepts?
- Do concepts represent objects, properties, events? Can you say? Are there concepts that are closely related?

3. DEFINITIONS
- Which concepts are defined? Which are not?
- Which concepts are defined explicitly? Which are implied?
- How much meaning needs to be inferred?
- Which concepts are defined specifically? Generally?
- Are there competing definitions for some concepts? Are there similar definitions for different concepts?
- Do any explicitly defined concepts not need definition?
- Are any concepts defined contrary to common convention?

4. RELATIONSHIPS
- What are the major relationships within the theory?
- Which relationships are obvious? Which are implied?
- Do relationships include all concepts? Which are not included?
- Are some concepts included in multiple relationships?

Continued

Box 4-1

Guide for the Description of Theory—cont'd

4. RELATIONSHIPS–cont'd

- Is there a hierarchy of relationships? Do relationships create meaning and understanding? Do they do this by describing, explaining? Predicting? What mix of each?
- Are relationships directional? What is their direction? Are they neutral?
- Are there mixed, competing, or incongruous relationships?
- Are relationships illustrated?

5. STRUCTURE

- How are overall and individual ideas organized?
- If outlined, what would the theory look like?
- Do relationships expand concepts into larger wholes or vice versa? Do they link concepts in a linear fashion?
- Does the structure move concepts away from or toward the purposes?
- Are there several structures that emerge? What is their form? Do they fit together?
- Could more than one structure represent the overall structural relationships?
- Where is there no structure?

6. ASSUMPTIONS

- What assumptions underlie the theory? Are assumptions explicit, implicit, or derivable from context and meanings?
- What are the individual, nurse, society, environment, and health assumed to be like?
- Do assumptions have an obvious value orientation? What is it?
- Could assumptions be factually verified?
- Where are assumptions located within the structure—prior to, within, or following theoretic reasoning?
- Can assumptions be hierarchically arranged or otherwise ordered?
- Do assumptions have any identifiable relationship to theoretic relationships or structure?
- Are there competing assumptions?

---

summarizes the questions that can be asked to form a complete description of theory. All questions are not necessarily answerable for a single theory. But, as you answer the questions that apply to the theory under consideration, concepts will be tentatively identified and the purpose of the theory will emerge. As definitions become evident, you will begin to see relationships. From the nature of the relationships, you will be able to address questions concerning the structure of the theory. Responses to questions concerning assumptions provide a level of awareness of meanings and will help you form an understanding of the theory. After an initial description of components, each component can be re-examined and revised.

For any theory, it is often not easy to describe theoretic purpose and assumptions. Concepts and their definitions may be more readily identifiable, especially if they are fairly explicit. Discerning relationships and structure is often a problematic area in describing theory, but these traits, too, will be present in theory.

Forming a complete description of theory requires systematic and critical examination of the work. Often every word, phrase, and sentence must be examined and re-examined for meaning. Ideas that emerge in response to the descriptive questions often lead to uncertainty and revisions of earlier ideas. After a time the description does begin to take shape, and fewer changes occur. There will always be some tentativeness in your descriptions because your description requires your own interpretive insights with respect to the theorist's ideas, and these insights change. If you are not able to reach a tentative resolution with respect to the fundamental nature of a theory after reasonable study and thought, the best course of action is to propose your ideas for revision and further development of the theory. Your continuing uncertainty indicates that further theoretic development must occur. Box 4-1 summarizes the questions that form a complete guide to the description of theory.

HOW DOES IT WORK? THE CRITICAL REFLECTION OF THEORY

Once theory is described, critical questions can be addressed to develop information about how well a theory might work for given purposes. Note that describing and critically reflecting theory are fundamentally different processes. Description can be compared with a more objective process of setting forth facts about the theory by asking, What is this? Critical reflection, by contrast, involves ascertaining how well a theory serves some purpose. In the section that follows, we identify questions that can be used in critical reflection. As you question how a theory works, you will form insights that will help you know how theory might be used and how it might be further developed.

As you study and read different nursing theories, you may think, "This does not seem right," "Maybe I could do this," or "This is really exciting." When these types of thoughts occur, you are comparing the theory with some personal and perhaps unrecognized ideas about what is important for theory. Each nurse's ideas of the adequacy of a theory are influenced by a personal perspective of what is valuable or good. For research, you might agree, "This could be helpful." For practice, you might think, "Maybe I could use this." For idea stimulation, you might think, "This really gives me some exciting new ideas." In these instances, you have formed an impression of the value of the theory from your personal values about practice, research, and critical thinking. Your values are important components that are integrated into a more formal critical reflection process.

Critical reflection contributes to understanding how well the theory relates to practice, research, or educational activities. Members of a discipline form ideas about what questions to ask and what responses are generally accepted if a theory is to be seen as valuable for the discipline. Just as there are many ways to describe theory, there are many critical questions that can be asked about the functional value of theory and many responses to these questions. Once the questions are asked, members of a discipline can consider what responses they tend to value and why. The questions we pose are consistent with generally accepted methods for evaluating theories that have been described in the nursing literature (Ellis, 1968; Fawcett, 1993; Hardy, 1974; Stevens-Barnum, 1998). However, our approach differs from accepted methods in that normative criteria are not implied.

The questions for critical reflection are as follows:

- How clear is this theory?
- How simple is this theory?
- How general is this theory?
- How accessible is this theory?
- How important is this theory?

Because these criteria are not normative, there are no correct answers to these questions, and the questions do not imply the responses. For example, How clear is this? does not necessarily mean that a theory should be perfectly clear. Rather, the people who address the question use it as a tool to focus on issues of clarity and gain understanding of how they might contribute to the theory's function for a particular purpose. As you engage in discussions that are centered around the questions, you can form a consensus with your colleagues as to where to go next with the theory. These insights can best be formed in discussion among people with diverse perspectives. For example, even though a theory that challenges assumptions about practice is somewhat unclear, it may be an important theory for changing nursing practice and for providing new concepts with which to work. The fact that it is not perfectly clear leaves room for imaging new possibilities, which may be part of the theory's strength.

Although each of the five critical reflection questions is fundamentally different, they are interrelated. For example, one question addresses accessibility, and another addresses generality. If a theory is seen as general or broad in scope, it may be less accessible (less related to empiric reality) than a narrower (less general) theory.

Responses to the questions used in creating a description affect your responses to the critical reflection questions. For example, to decide how clear, accessible, or general a theory is, you need to describe the purpose of the theory, what concepts are included, and how they are structured. As your description of theory is formed, you can begin the process of critical reflection. The ideas you develop from this process contribute to your own critical insights and to substantive discussion that gives direction for further theory development. The questions for critically reflecting theory are described in the following sections.

How Clear Is This Theory?

In determining how clear a theory is, you will be considering semantic clarity, semantic consistency, structural clarity, and structural consistency. Clarity, in general, refers to how well the theory can be understood and how consistently the ideas are conceptualized. Semantic clarity and consistency primarily refer to the understandability of theoretic meaning as it relates to concepts. Structural clarity and consistency reflect the understandability of connections between concepts within the theory and the whole of the theory.

Semantic Clarity. The definitions of concepts in the theory are an important aspect of semantic clarity. Definitions help to establish empiric meaning for concepts within the theory. If concepts are not defined or are incompletely defined, the empiric indicators for the idea become less clear. When concepts are clearly defined, identification of empiric indicators is relatively easy. Clarity implies, in part, that when different nurses read the theory, a similar empiric reality comes to mind when the word for the concept is used. If there are no definitions or if only a few of the concepts are defined, clarity is limited.

The types of definitions that are used within theory affect semantic clarity. Definitions that reflect both specific and general traits enhance clarity, whereas a general or a specific definition alone often limits clarity. Specific definitions lend clarity because they provide clear and accurate guidance for the intended empiric indicators for a concept; general definitions contribute a contextual sense of meaning for concepts and lend a richness of meaning that is not possible when concepts are specifically defined. Considering the extent to which each type of definition contributes to clarity of meaning can help you form your own ideas about the adequacy of the theory for your purpose.

Clarity may be obscured by borrowing terms from other disciplines or by using common-language terms that carry broad general meanings. Words like *stress* and *coping* have general common-language meanings, and they also have specific theoretic meanings in other disciplines. If words with multiple meanings are used in theory and not defined, a person's everyday meaning of the term, rather than what is meant in the theory, is often assumed; therefore, clarity is lost. Clarity is enhanced when the concept's definition is consistent with common meanings of the term within the profession.

Clarity is affected when words that have no common meaning are used or when the theorist invents or coins words to represent some idea. Coined words can help to convey a meaning for which there is no word, but they can also detract from clarity, especially when a more familiar word or phrase would suffice. It would be possible to generate an entire theory about quizzendroids, plankerods, and ziots. The theory could be logical and consistent but unclear because the words are invented and have no meaning. Although this example is exaggerated, it demonstrates the effects on clarity when vague or strange words are used, when words are not defined, or when words with many possible meanings are used and not defined.

Semantic clarity can also be affected by excessive verbiage. Normally, varying words to represent similar meanings is a writing skill that can be used to avoid overuse of a single term. But, in theory, if several similar concepts are used interchangeably when one would suffice, there is excess verbiage, and the clarity of the theory's presentation is reduced rather than improved. In theory, varying the word for important concepts interjects subtly different meanings. For example, interchanging the words *restoration, rehabilitation,* and *recovery* for the same concept changes clarity because each word has a slightly different meaning and suggests different contexts of use.

Clarity is also affected when excessive narrative is included. Semantic clarity may be decreased by excessive examples; however, the judicious use of examples usually aids clarity. Diagrams can enhance or obscure clarity. To enhance clarity, diagrams should be self-explanatory and simple in expression because overly complex illustrations discourage comprehension. In general, the alternate mode of providing information in the form of diagrams helps to make the ideas in the theory clearer.

Economy of words, key definitions, and wise use of examples and diagrams lend clarity. Absolute semantic clarity can never be achieved, nor is it necessarily desirable. Because of the limitations of language, no matter how clearly the theorist represents theoretic meaning, it will not be perceived uniformly by all readers.

Semantic Consistency. Semantic consistency is a second feature to consider with respect to the question of clarity. A theory that is inconsistently presented leads to confusion. Semantic consistency means that the concepts of the theory are used in ways that are consistent with their definition. Sometimes a definition is explicitly stated, and somewhere within the theory another meaning is implied. When key words are not explicitly defined, their implied meanings may be inconsistent from one usage to the next. Occasionally, words are explicitly defined but in different ways. Inconsistencies that occur when terms are defined explicitly are fairly easy to uncover, but other types of inconsistencies may be more covert.

The consistent use of basic assumptions is important in achieving consistency. The theory's purpose, definitions of concepts, and relationships need to be consistent with the stated assumptions of the theory. Examples and diagrams can also be considered in light of the assumptions of the theory. Suppose, for example, a basic theoretic assumption is the unity of persons and environment and that both change simultaneously and irreversibly through time and space. This assumption is consistent with a definition of *health* as expanding consciousness but inconsistent with a theoretic conceptualization of health as a state of adaptation. Adaptation typically implies conforming or adjusting to environmental stimuli in order to fit within the environment. The concept of adaptation tends to suggest the assumption that events external to the person are primary as a determinant of health and that the person and the environment are separate entities. Unity of person and environment is a concept that can be used to convey an assumption that humans and environment are interconnected and change simultaneously. Simultaneous change negates the idea of conforming or adjusting to stimuli as health; rather, it implies incorporating change, becoming a different person, and increasing options and awareness of choice.

For clarity, the purposes of the theory must be consistent with all other components. A purpose of health, achieved by deliberate nursing actions, may be at odds with the basic assumption that health is deterministic. The purpose in this example is to create something that is assumed to be deterministic and therefore cannot be influenced by deliberate acts. Becoming aware of this inconsistency helps to clarify other meanings that are conveyed in the definitions and other components of the theory.

In reflecting on consistency, examine your descriptions for each component of theory and consider where there are consistencies and inconsistencies within the descriptive elements of the theory, as well as between them. Definitions must be examined for consistency with each other and in relation to assumptions. Structure is sometimes inconsistent with relationships. If a theory is extremely inconsistent, it is difficult to continue the process of critical reflection concerning the theory. Some semantic inconsistencies within theory are more common early in their development and leave room for new possibilities for further development. However, inconsistencies at the basic roots of theory, such as between assumptions and goals, have implications that will affect the entire theory and must be addressed.

Structural Clarity. Structural clarity is closely linked to semantic clarity. Structural clarity refers to how understandable the connections and reasoning within theory are. The descriptive elements of structure and relationships provide important information for addressing this dimension of clarity.

In a theory with structural clarity, you can readily recognize the underlying conceptual network. With structural clarity, concepts are interconnected and organized into a coherent whole. If you cannot discern the structure of the theory, you begin to search for those structural elements that are related and for gaps that occur in the flow of the theory. If all major relationships are included within a single structure, clarity is enhanced. Clarity is lost if the relationships are not contained within a coherent structure. Pieces of relationships, rudiments of structure, or concepts that stand alone are evidence that parts have not yet been integrated into the whole during the development of the theory.

Structural Consistency. Structural consistency relates to the use of different structural forms within theory. Usually theory is built around one predominant structural form. Sometimes one form provides the general profile for the conception of the relationships of theory, and subcomponents of the theory take a somewhat different form. Whatever the structure, consistency throughout the theory with respect to the structure serves as a conceptual map that enhances clarity. A theorist may begin with a structural movement that is linear. If this structure is reflected in the relationships as the theory develops, you will observe a high level of structural consistency. A shift in reasoning to a structure that integrates and coalesces concepts may be confusing, or the reasoning might function well within the overall structure.

In summary, How clear is this theory? can be asked to explore in what ways a theory is clear and comprehensible, how it is not, and what its level of clarity means for the development and use of the theory. The ideas of semantic and structural consistency and clarity can be used to guide discussion of issues of clarity. A very general (broad-scope) theory may be quite ambiguous but useful in stimulating new ideas. A midrange theory of hopelessness, for example, may have aspects that are vague but still be important in helping nurses understand the experience. However, the ambiguity of that same theory may affect its usefulness for guiding research. Becoming aware of the ways in which clarity is obscured in light of your purpose makes it possible to design ways to further develop its clarity. The degree to which a theory must be clear depends on how the nurse intends to use it.

How Simple Is This Theory?

Simplicity means that the number of elements within each descriptive category, particularly concepts and their interrelationships, are minimal. Complexity implies many theoretic relationships between and among numerous concepts. The following example illustrates theoretic simplicity. Suppose that a theory contained three major concepts: *A*, *B*, and *C*. A theory interrelating these as discrete concepts would be quite simple because only three interrelationships would be possible: *A* and *B*, *A* and *C*, and *B* and *C*. Adding subconcepts 1 and 2 to *A*, *B*, and *C* (e.g., *A*1, *A*2) would leave the theorist with three major concepts (*A*, *B*, and *C*) and six subconcepts, for a total of nine. A theorist working with nine concepts has significantly greater theoretic complexity than a theorist working with only three concepts. Adding even one or two concepts to a theory greatly increases the potential for theoretic interrelationships and, subsequently, complexity.

The desirability of simplicity or complexity varies with the stage of theory development. In grounded theory, for example, there may be considerable complexity as the theory begins to emerge, but, as it develops, relationships and concepts are coalesced, and the theory becomes more simple. Regardless of the approach to theory development, some concepts created early in the process may eventually be deleted or changed. In the previous example, suppose concepts *A*, *A*1, and *A*2 came to be seen as unimportant in relation to the theory's purpose. The theoretic complexity added by *A* and its subconcepts could be removed, and only the simpler relationships between *B* and *C* and their subconcepts would remain.

Theories reflect varying degrees of simplicity. In nursing, some situations suggest the need for relatively simple and broad theory that can be used as a general guide for practice. Other situations suggest simple but more empirically accessible theory to guide research. Still other situations suggest the need for theory that is relatively complex because of the value such theory has for enhancing understanding of extremely complex practice situations.

How General Is This Theory?

The generality of a theory refers to its breadth of scope and purpose; a general theory can be applied to a broad array of situations. *Parsimony* is sometimes used as a synonym to describe the trait of theoretic simplicity, but the concept of parsimony also includes the idea of generality. A parsimonious theory is conceptually simple (contains few structural elements) but accounts for a broad range of empiric experiences.

The scope of concepts and purposes within the theory provide clues to its generality. A theory containing broad concepts will encompass more ideas with fewer words than one containing very narrow concepts. Concepts of humans and universe could be interpreted as organizing almost every fact or idea possible. A comprehensive theory with these two concepts would be highly general. A theory interrelating the individual and the physical environment is less general, although still fairly broad in scope. The concept of individual implies that the theory is concerned with a single person. The use of *physical* as a modifier for environment conveys the notion of environment in part only. Information about individuals in communities could not be understood within this theory. A theory relating characteristics of acutely ill people with the intensive care unit environment is even less general, and the scope of concepts narrows.

Questions that address the generality of theory include the following: To whom does this theory apply, and when does it apply? Does the purpose pertain to all health care professionals? To people in general? Does the purpose apply to specific specialties of nursing and only at given times? The more limited the scope of application of the theory, the less general the theory.

Whether generality is viewed as desirable depends on your purpose for the theory. General theory organizes many ideas and is quite useful for generating ideas or hypotheses. Nursing theories that address broad concepts, such as individuals, society, health, and environment, have a high degree of generality and are useful for organizing ideas about universal health behaviors. Theories that address a specific human experience such as pain are less general and, because of their relative specificity, are useful for guiding practice in a clinical setting.

How Accessible Is This Theory?

Accessibility addresses the extent to which empiric indicators can be identified for concepts within the theory and how attainable the projected outcomes of the theory are. If a theory is to be used for explaining some aspect of the practice world, its theoretic concepts must be linked to empiric indicators available in practice.

Only selected dimensions of highly abstract concepts may be empirically accessible. If the concepts of a theory do not reflect empiric dimensions or if the empiric dimensions are very obscure, they may be ideas that cannot be explored or understood empirically.

Consider the example of a theory about rehabilitation and interaction. The theoretic definitions of the concepts are clues to the accessibility of the theory. Without definition, the words *rehabilitation* and *interaction* can assume many dimensions of meaning. If the concepts are defined, how they are to be empirically accessed is clearer. If definitions do not clearly suggest their empiric basis and the purpose of the theory is to promote rehabilitation, an empiric basis for rehabilitation must be located within a clinical context.

Increasing the complexity within theories often increases empiric accessibility. As subconceptual categories are clarified, empiric indicators become more precise. Suppose that the concepts of rehabilitation and interaction are related within the same theory. The theory is judged to have a high degree of generality and simplicity because the concepts are broad and few in number. Complexity would be increased by designating five subconcepts for each. Those five subconcepts are likely to have more precise empiric bases than the broader concepts. With empirically accessible subconcepts, the empiric accessibility of the theory increases. If a concept does not have an empiric basis at the outset, specifying subconcepts for larger wholes does not increase empiric accessibility.

Research testing both requires and establishes the empiric accessibility of concepts. For example, if rehabilitation is defined operationally in a research project as "able to complete activities of daily living independently," you have established a clear link between the idea—rehabilitation—and a reasonable clinical observation. If the research supports the hypothesis derived from the theory, it also provides evidence of empiric accessibility for the concept of rehabilitation.

Empiric accessibility of concepts contained within theory is basic to validating theoretic relationships and using the theory in practice. Although grounded approaches to generating theory assume empiric accessibility, the extent to which empiric accessibility is important can vary. Considering what the theory is developed to do will help you make judgments about how empirically accessible a theory should be. Theory that provides a conceptual perspective of clinical practice may not need much empiric accessibility. If a theory is to be used to guide research, empiric accessibility is important. If a theory is to be used to shape nursing practice, concepts need to be empirically accessible in the clinical area. If concepts are not empirically grounded, creating conceptual meaning may provide direction for empiric indicators needed for research.

How Important Is This Theory?

In nursing, the importance of a theory is closely tied to the idea of its clinical significance or practical value. An important theory is forward-looking, useful, and valuable for creating a desired future. The central question is, Does the theory create a reality that is important to nursing? Many realities will be important to nursing. Some nursing theory guides research and practice, some generates radically new ideas about health and caring, and some differentiates the focus of nursing from other service professions.

If a theory contains concepts, definitions, purposes, and assumptions that are grounded in practice, it will have practical value for enhancing theory-based research. A theory that has limited empiric accessibility may not have practical value for research but can stimulate ideas and spark political action that improves practice.

One approach to addressing the question of importance is to reflect on the theory's basic theoretic assumptions. If underlying assumptions are unsound, the importance of the theory is minimal. If, for example, a theory is based on a view of the individual as parts, its importance for nursing is minimal. If a theory is based on an assumption of wholism and it moves understanding of wholism to a new dimension, it is likely to be highly important to nursing.

Theories that have extremely broad purposes may be essentially unattainable and therefore have limited value for creating clinical outcomes. This same theory may be important for generating ideas and challenging practice.

The importance of theory depends on the professional and personal values of the person who is addressing the question. Asking the questions, Do I like this theory? and Why? will help you identify the values you hold for yourself, your practice, the profession, and the theory. Contributing your ideas about what is important for nursing through careful deliberation and discussion among nurse colleagues will help discern the direction for a theory to achieve important professional purposes.

Forming a Complete Critical Reflection

In summary, the five questions for critically reflecting a description of theory are as follows:

1. *Is this clear?* This question addresses the clarity and consistency of presentation. Clarity and consistency may be both semantic and structural.
2. *Is this simple?* This question addresses the number of structural components and relationships within theory. Complexity implies

numerous relational components within theory; simplicity implies fewer relational components.

3. *Is this general?* This question addresses the scope of experiences covered by theory. Generality infers a wide scope of phenomena, whereas specificity narrows the range of events included in theory. Generality combined with simplicity yields parsimony.

4. *Is this accessible?* This question addresses the extent to which concepts within the theory are grounded in empirically identifiable phenomena.

5. *Is this important?* This question addresses the extent to which theory leads to valued nursing goals in practice, research, and education.

The summary of critical reflection questions presented in Box 4-2 provides a guide for forming a critical reflection of theory.

Box 4-2
Guide for the Critical Reflection of Theory

HOW CLEAR IS THIS THEORY?

- Are major concepts defined?
- Are significant concepts not defined? Are definitions clear? Congruent? Consistent?
- Are words coined? Are coined words defined?
- Are words borrowed from other disciplines and used differently in this context?
- Is the amount of explanation appropriate? Too much? Not enough?
- Are examples or diagrams helpful? Not helpful? Needed and not present?
- Are the examples and diagrams used meaningful?
- Are basic assumptions consistent with one another? With purposes?
- Is the view of person and environment compatible?
- Are the same terms defined differently?
- Are different terms defined similarly?
- Are concepts used in a manner consistent with their definition?
- Are diagrams and examples consistent with the text?
- Are compatible and coherent structures suggested for different parts of the theory?
- Can the theory be followed? Can an overall structure be diagrammed?
- Where, if any, are gaps in the flow? Do all concepts fit within the theory?
- Are there any ambiguities as a result of sequence of presentation?
- Does the theorist accomplish what she or he sets out to do?

Continued

Box 4-2
Guide for the Critical Reflection of Theory—cont'd

HOW SIMPLE IS THIS THEORY?

- How many relationships are contained within the theory?
- How are the relationships organized?
- How many concepts are contained in the theory?
- Are some concepts differentiated into subconcepts and others not?
- Can concepts be combined without losing theoretic meaning?
- Is the theory complex in some areas and not in others?
- Does the theory tend to describe, explain, or predict? Impart understanding? Create meaning?

HOW GENERAL IS THIS THEORY?

- How specific are the purposes of this theory? Do they apply to all or only some practice areas? When?
- Is this theory specific to nursing? If not, who else could use it? Why?
- Is the purpose justifiably a nursing purpose?
- If subpurposes exist, do they reflect nursing actions? How broad are the concepts within the theory?

HOW ACCESSIBLE IS THIS THEORY?

- Are the concepts broad or narrow?
- How specific or general are definitions within the theory?
- Are the concepts' empiric indicators identifiable in reality? Are they within the realm of nursing?
- Do the definitions provided for the concepts adequately reflect their meanings?
- Is a very narrow definition offered for a broad concept? A broad meaning for a narrow concept?
- If words are coined, are they defined?

HOW IMPORTANT IS THIS THEORY?

- Does the theory have potential to influence nursing actions? If so, to what end? Is that end desirable?
- Does the theory influence nursing education? Nursing research? If so, to what end? Is that end desirable?
- How specific are the purposes of the theory? Do they provide a general framework within which to act or a means to predict phenomena?
- Is the theory's position about people, about nursing, and about the environment consistent with nursing's philosophy?
- Given the purpose of the theory and its orientation, what of significance for nursing or health care has been omitted?
- Is the stated or implied purpose one that is important to nursing? Why?
- Will use of the theory help or hinder nursing in any way? If so, how?
- Will application of this theory resolve any important issues in nursing? Will it resolve any problems?
- Is the theory futuristic and forward-looking?
- Will research based on the theory answer important questions?
- Are the concepts within the domain of nursing?
- Do I like this theory? Why?

CONCLUSION

Description and critical reflection of theory can be used by nurses for a variety of reasons. By asking, What is this and how does it work? practitioners can make decisions about using theories in practice. Researchers and other scholars can make appropriate research decisions. Educators can determine how well the theory serves the purposes of nursing education. Overall, the process of careful reasoned description and critical reflection is easily accessible and can guide the development of theory so that it is in harmony with an envisioned future.

Reference List

Abdellah FG: *Patient-centered approaches to nursing,* New York, 1960, Macmillan.

Ellis R: Characteristics of significant theories, *Nurs Res* 17:217, 1968.

Fawcett J: *Analysis and evaluation of conceptual models of nursing,* ed 2, Philadelphia, 1993, FA Davis.

Hall LE: Another view of nursing care and quality. In Straub KM, Parker KS, editors: *Continuity in patient care: the role of nursing,* Washington, DC, 1966, Catholic University Press.

Hardy ME: Theories: components, development, evaluation, *Nurs Res* 23:100, 1974.

Koltoff NJ: The use of the laboratory, *Nurs Res* 16:122, 1967.

Stevens-Barnum BJ: *Nursing theory,* ed 5, Boston, 1998, Lippincott-Raven.

Chapter 5

Replicating and Validating Empiric Knowledge Using Research

Research extends knowledge through application of scientific methods—not with absolute certainty—but with minimal misinformation. Skepticism, alert self criticism, constant testing of hypotheses by empirical research and awareness of limitations of science make research a most dependable source of information.

Laurie M. Gunter (1964, p. 231)

In this chapter we focus on methods for replicating and validating empiric phenomena by using research methods. Figure 5-1 shows the empiric quadrant of our model for nursing knowledge development, highlighting the role of replicating and validating theories and models. These processes authenticate what is expressed in the formal knowledge of the discipline, which in turn strengthens scientific competence in practice. Replication and validation of theories and models also draw on practice-based methods, which we present in Chapter 6.

Development of empiric knowledge depends on formal processes of verification that use systematic methods of research. Research can be used as a means to test theoretic relationships and as a method to generate concepts or relationships for the construction of theory. Philosophic commitments of researchers, the philosophy of nursing, and the emerging theory are integral to the choices the researcher makes about method. Deliberate choices that link research methods, theory, and practice are basic to developing sound empiric knowledge.

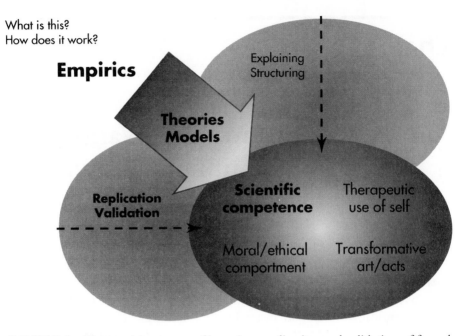

FIGURE 5-1 The empiric pattern of knowing: replication and validation of formal expressions of empiric knowledge.

Of all of the processes of empiric knowledge development, research-related activities are more visible to the casual observer than the cognitively based theoretic processes. The concept of research is often associated with the image of a laboratory where experiments are conducted or some other activity occurs that involves discovering facts. Actually, creating empiric knowledge is more related to abstract theoretic processes than it is to uncovering isolated facts that can be reported in great detail and with numbers. Factual knowledge is useful, but facts alone are insufficient for developing empiric knowledge. To develop empiric knowledge, facts must be interpreted in relation to one another and conceived as having meaning (Bleich, 1978; Greer, 1969; Scheffler, 1967; Silva and Rothbart, 1984).

In this chapter we focus on theory as a primary form of empirics because theory is usually structured in a way that forms links with scientific research methods. Broadly speaking, any discursively presented form of knowledge that is capable of empiric replication and validation is an empiric knowledge form. Validation may not depend on traditional research methods but could consist of examining the extent of correspondence between one work and another. For example, a historical analysis or a critical theoretical analysis would not be validated with traditional scientific research methods, but they could be validated by comparing these works to other works addressing the same period or the same sociopolitical dynamic. Facts, conceptual models, descriptions, and frameworks—all forms of empiric knowledge expression— can provide direction for replication and validation with a wide variety of empiric methods.

In the next section we distinguish between theory-linked and isolated research. The remainder of the chapter reviews the processes required to refine concepts and theoretic relationships with empiric research methods, and we review approaches that assure that any given research project fulfills sound standards of theoretic adequacy.

THEORY-LINKED RESEARCH AND ISOLATED RESEARCH

Research, like theorizing, can be conducted in a variety of ways and with multiple motivating factors. There are many descriptions of different types of research, and each research text presents a somewhat different way of viewing the total process. The traits in common for each approach reflect certain basic standards that have been established to obtain results that are considered reliable (consistent, undistorted) and valid (accurately representative of empiric reality).

Two types of research can be conducted: theory-linked or isolated research. The major trait that distinguishes theory-linked research from isolated research is that theory-linked research is designed to develop, refine, or test theory. This quality sets the stage for the study to contribute to the larger knowledge of the discipline. Isolated research, by contrast, is not linked to the processes of theory development.

From a research point of view, theory-linked and isolated research can both be of excellent quality. Both types of research can ultimately contribute to knowledge, although isolated research is much more limited in the contribution it can make to a discipline. Because theory-linked research is conceived and conducted to create, examine, or extend theory, the findings of research imply significance at an abstract level of understanding, opening potential to explore different avenues of possibility.

In isolated research, the investigator formulates questions or hypotheses and uses accepted methods to refute or support the hypotheses or to answer the questions. Questions or hypotheses may come from the practical circumstances surrounding the investigator's work, the imagination, an idea that occurred as the investigator read other research results, or any number of other sources. These same factors can also provide direction for the development of theory-linked research.

All research is confined to a particular place and a time in history. Because theories are constructions of the mind, they can transcend, to a certain extent, the limitations of time and space. The cultural and historical circumstances of the theorist influence the mental construction of the theory, but because the theory is an abstraction, it is possible to move beyond the limits of particular circumstances. Isolated research, which often focuses on the particulars of a specific problem, offers little potential for speculating about the significance of the research beyond what can be justified by the method, design, and analysis of study results. The results of isolated research can provide new insights that prompt the researcher, or someone reading the report of the research, to speculate about larger implications of the research for the discipline, which in turn can lead to developing theory that has broader meaning for the discipline.

Theory-linked research has advantages that overcome the limitations of the specific place and time in which the research occurs. Theory-linked research hypotheses that are developed from abstract statements of the theory represent a translation of the theory's abstract statements to the circumstances of the specific study. These research findings can be generalized only within limits, just as those reported in isolated research. However, the study findings in theory-linked research can be retranslated to theoretic terms and implications discussed in relation to the theory.

Problems of Theory-Linked Research

Although theory-linked research has definite advantages over isolated research in its ability to contribute to the development of knowledge, certain hazards and problems are unique to this type of research.

Inappropriate Use of Theories. It is possible to use a theory inappropriately in conducting research. For example, if a theory is designed to explain animal behavior, it may not be appropriate as a basis for explaining human behavior, and vice versa, without sufficient conceptual examination. Theory and theoretic concepts that are used inappropriately lead to erroneous conclusions. Reed (1978), for example, describes how some theories in behavioral sciences have resulted in erroneous information concerning primate behavior. Using theories of human behavior, researchers have categorized primate sexual behavior as either monogamous or polygamous. On the basis of limited observations of animal behavior, it became common practice to describe animal behavior by these terms. Reed (1978, p. 49) points out that, in reality, animals seldom cohabit on the basis of sex differences, and segregation of male and female primates is more pronounced than cohabitation. Theories sometimes provide a mental set that clouds observations, especially if the theory is assumed to be true or consistent with prevailing values.

Theories as Barriers. Theories can obscure a researcher's ability to notice certain features or events. The mind-set provided by theory, whether appropriate or not, may preclude recognition of other possibilities. When the focus is on expected outcomes, unless something startling or drastically different occurs, some elements may not be noticed. For example, you can view a child's behavior and, because of a certain theory, assume that what you observe is problem-solving ability. At the same time, you might fail to notice other things about the child's behavior that are not brought to your attention by the theory. These other behaviors might include less obvious and therefore easily overlooked actions such as body posture, facial expressions, or eye motion. It is possible that qualities of these behaviors relate to problem-solving ability, but the mental set that you acquire from the theory focuses your attention on limited behaviors, and something potentially important in understanding the child's reality is overlooked.

Paradoxically, although a theory may be useful and appropriate for understanding reality, it may limit your thinking about the range of possibilities and experiences. Overcoming this difficulty requires you to constantly question what you read, think, and observe. Theory is not intended to represent exact truth or reality; it is intended to be an approximation and a tool to see new possibilities. The purpose for using research to develop theory is to discover to what extent a theory can be regarded as sound and to what extent it functions to open new possibilities.

Ethical Considerations. Theories can also exceed acceptable limits of reality; theories as mental constructions may relate ideas that cannot or should not be tested, out of respect for human and animal rights and dignity. For example, given the threat of nuclear accidents, you might imagine that it would be useful to predict events in a large population of people who experience a significant exposure to radiation. This knowledge might help in preparing for this circumstance. In reality, it is not ethical to subject humans or animals to such an experience to develop theory. It is also not feasible to test imagined theoretic ideas that claim to predict the consequences of exposure to radiation. Ethical considerations may also be much subtler and need to be examined. For example, certain approaches to the study of cultures outside the mainstream (for example, differently-abled women, ethnic minority groups, gay or lesbian cultures) undermine those cultures and provide avenues for further discrimination.

Occasionally, historical circumstances provide evidence that is used to develop useful theory, but further testing is limited by concern for human and animal welfare. Theories of mother-infant attachment and separation grew out of the experiences of wartime children separated from their mothers for extended periods of time. The evidence that grew out of the historical disaster was amply sufficient to demonstrate the harmful effects, and further research that replicates similar circumstances is ethically indefensible.

REFINING CONCEPTS AND THEORETIC RELATIONSHIPS

A particular type of theory-linked research is that designed specifically to refine concepts and theoretic relationships. These types of investigations are crucial early in the stages of a theory's development but can be used at any point of theoretic development. Refining concepts and theoretic relationships involves a focus on the correspondence of the ideas of the theory with accessible experience (Dubin, 1978; Glaser and Strauss, 1967; Newman, 1979; Reynolds, 1971). Because empiric concepts and theories are abstractions of what can be observed in experience, a translation is made from the theoretic to the empiric (deductive approach) and from the empiric to the theoretic (inductive approach).

To function as viable structural elements of theory, concepts require empiric validation to assure their adequacy in representing actual human experience. Descriptive approaches, both quantitative and qualitative, are typically used to obtain empiric evidence that the concepts, as created within the theoretic structure, have adequate empiric referents and operational definitions. The evidence from the investigations may point to needed conceptual shifts to better represent the experience. Investigations designed to develop and refine empiric indicators and operational definitions for concepts are crucial for adequate research to refine and test theoretic relationships.

Theoretic relationships, which connect two or more concepts in a specific structure, depend on the empiric adequacy of the concepts themselves. The activities of refining concepts and theoretic relationships involve both qualitative and quantitative approaches. Replication is repeating the validation activities in other contexts. Theoretic relationships cannot be proven, but it is possible to show empiric support for the proposed relationships. If the evidence does not support theoretic relationships, the ideas of the theory cannot be sustained as theory. Alternative theoretic explanations are then considered, based on the empiric evidence.

Refining concepts and theoretic relationships draws on one or more subcomponents: (1) validating empiric indicators for the concepts, (2) empirically grounding emerging relationships, and (3) validating relationships through empiric methods.

Validating Empiric Indicators

Empiric indicators and operational definitions are used to represent concepts as variables in empiric research and are empirically formed for concepts arising from inductive approaches. Formally structured theory can propose empiric indicators, but, until they are put into operation in research, they remain speculative. Using the ideas in actual research makes it possible to refine the ideas of the theory.

Consider the following abstract relationship statement:

> As the adult's eye contact increases, the infant's eye contact will increase.

A research project is designed to obtain empiric evidence about the use of eye contact as an empiric indicator of mothering. Details such as length of gaze and frequency of eye contact are specified for the relatively abstract concept of "eye contact." To use these indicators, the researcher creates a method for observing and timing the length of gaze and the frequency of eye contact.

Part of the process for identifying empiric indicators, especially when primarily deductive processes are used, is to state operational definitions. Operational definitions specify the standards or criteria to be used in making the observations. For example, an operational definition of the term *gaze* might be "a steady, direct, visual focusing on an object that lasts at least 3 seconds." This definition indicates what *gaze* is (the empiric indicator for visual contact), characteristics that are to be used in calling a behavior a gaze (direct visual focusing on an object), and a standard time parameter that distinguishes a gaze from other related behaviors such as a glance or a look.

It is more difficult to refine empiric indicators for concepts that are more abstract than the concept of eye contact. Many concepts related to nursing (for example, anxiety, body image, and self-esteem) are highly abstract and cannot be directly measured. Tests and tools have been constructed to provide an indirect estimate of traits such as these. The fact that they cannot be measured directly does not mean they are nonexistent or cannot be assessed. The empiric challenge is to refine ideas about and evidence for empiric indicators so that estimates of relationships can be explored.

The difficulties of finding adequate empiric indicators for abstract concepts can be compared to trying to describe what a tomato tastes like. Once a person bites a tomato, that person knows how it tastes. The descriptions of that taste are not at all adequate in comparison with the actual taste experience. When we turn to many of the concepts that are important for nursing, then even the actual experience is not as clearly perceived as the experience of tasting a tomato, and the problems of finding reliable empiric indicators becomes even more complex and difficult. For example, anxiety is an abstract concept that can be theoretically defined, but when we turn to explore the experience of anxiety, we find that people recognize what we mean by the term *anxiety* but that their actual experiences are as elusive as the taste of a tomato, and the experience of anxiety is not as clearly perceived as the perception of a taste. However, if the concept is important for nursing, empiric knowledge development depends on diligent efforts to specify as accurately as possible the link between the abstract concept and the actual human experience. These examples underscore the value of concept development for adequate theory in nursing.

One approach that can be used to derive empiric measures for abstract nursing concepts is to use multiple empiric indicators to form operational definitions. For example, anxiety might be measured with a self-report tool. The tool can be constructed to include many sensations that are generally indicative of anxiety. The operational definition of the concept of anxiety then becomes what is assessed with the use of the tool. Anxiety might also be empirically assessed by observing a person's behavior and the physiologic indicators of neuroendocrine function. The operational definitions would include specific ways to measure the behaviors observed and the specific range of laboratory test results associated with anxiety. All of these empiric indicators are possible. If they are used together in situations in which anxiety is likely to occur, the study will provide substantive evidence about the usefulness of each measure as an empiric indicator.

When inductive research processes form the basis for refining empiric indicators, the indicators are directly or indirectly observed and are used to form concepts. Knowing the empiric indicators used in generating the concepts would assist the deductive testing and extension of the theory into other contexts.

The work of Ferrans (1997; Ferrans and Powers, 1992) and her colleagues in developing the idea of "quality of life" is one example of the use of several different research approaches to develop and refine a conceptual model. "Quality of life" can be seen as a large construct that is subsumed by several other conceptual elements. Ferrans used qualitative research methods to find out what indicators people from different cultural groups associated with the idea of quality of life. They also used factor analysis techniques to find clusters among the various perceptions that emerged from their research. They identified four domains of quality of life: health and functioning, psychologic-spiritual, social and economic, and family. They then developed a tool, the Quality of Life Index, to operationalize the concept of quality of life and its subconcepts.

Empirically Grounding Emerging Relationships

The process of empirically grounding emerging relationships involves connecting experiences with representations of those experiences. When an abstract theoretic relationship is taken as the starting point, the investigator designs a study in which the hypothetic relationship, framed in terms of the operational definitions of concepts, can be studied. Several investigations are required to confirm that the relationship proposed is accurate. When the investigations provide sufficient empiric evidence to draw conclusions about the relationship, the investigator can return to the theoretic ideas and refine the theoretic statements to reflect what has been supported empirically. These conclusions are often presented as examples, citing the empiric investigations, within the narrative explanations of the theory.

An investigator can begin by exploring a selected empiric situation as the starting point, with the goal to find the concepts and relationships that accurately represent a situation that is not yet clearly understood but is recognized as important to the discipline of nursing. The investigator selects a social context in which the phenomenon under consideration is likely to occur and observes the interactions and circumstances of that context. From the observations the investigator derives relationship statements that are grounded in the available empiric evidence. A variety of inductive approaches can be used to ground emerging relationships (Glaser and Strauss, 1967; Lincoln and Guba, 1985).

Validating Relationships Through Empiric Methods

Validating theoretic relationships requires creating a design that tests the explanatory power of a designated relationship. Designs may be proposed after theory is structured (deduction) or may generate theory that, because of the design, is considered to be valid and ready for replication and validation in other settings (induction).

A key to deductive validation of theoretic relationships is to employ a design that ensures that the proposed relationship is actually the one that accounts for the study findings. For example, if a study concludes that a mother's gaze prompts an infant's gaze in return, the researcher needs to consider ways to be sure that it is actually the mother's gaze that accounts for the infant's behavior. Typically the researcher designs the study so that other factors that could influence the behavior of the infants in the study (for example, sensory experiences such as noise, touch, or visual distractions that might affect the process of visual interaction) are held constant or accounted for.

The purpose of deductively refining any relationship statement is to provide empiric evidence that the relationships proposed in the theory are adequate when represented in a specific situation. With each approach to design that is used, the research question or hypothesis is revised to suit the type of design selected. Empiric evidence based on many different approaches to research design provides a basis for judging the adequacy of the theory. If theoretic statements are deductively tested and not supported by empiric evidence, one or more of the following four possibilities can account for the disparity between the theory and empiric findings:

1. *The meaning of the concepts is not adequately created.* The process of creating conceptual meaning can be used to determine if the definitions and meanings of the concepts under study are clear and if they are well differentiated from related concepts. If they are not, theoretic revisions can be made, resulting in new approaches to empiric study.

2. *The relationship statement is not adequately structured.* The processes of theory structuring and contextualizing can be used to examine the logic or form of the statements. Given the benefit of the empiric evidence, new insights into the form and structure of the theory might emerge. The theorist can revise the theoretic relationship statements on the basis of these insights.

3. *The empiric indicators for the concept are not adequately named.* The empiric evidence might point to new possibilities for empiric indicators or suggest revisions in the existing indicators. This process is particularly important when the empiric indicators represent highly abstract concepts and are constructed out of speculative ideas about how the concepts can be observed empirically.

4. *The operational definitions are inadequate or inconsistent.* Typically, conflicting research results are attributed to faulty operational definitions and the related measurement problems of empiric research. This is a possibility, but accurate assessment depends on adequately conceived concepts, sound theoretic statements, and adequate empiric indicators. If these are all in place, it is then reasonable to consider problems in operationalization.

When inductive methods are used to refine concepts and theoretic relationships, the relationships may be considered valid if processes for generating them are done carefully. When relationships are deduced from inductively generated theory, they can be tested in similar settings or extended into new contexts. When this occurs, problems with faulty concepts, relational statements, empiric indicators, and operational definitions will become evident.

DESIGNING THEORETICALLY SOUND EMPIRIC RESEARCH

Investigations that are linked to theory can take one of two forms: theory-generating and theory-validating. In the following sections, we explain each type of approach and provide guidelines that can be used as a frame of reference for designing investigations in the planning or that can be used to assess the theoretic adequacy of a completed investigation.

Theory-Generating Research

Research that generates theory is designed to generate and describe relationships without imposing preconceived notions of what these phenomena mean. This approach is usually thought of as inductive. It is impossible to observe events in the real world without some preconceived mental image of what they mean. Pre-existing mental images are inherent in the experience of being socialized in a human culture; the process of learning the theories of a discipline conveys meanings. A researcher who designs a study to generate theory observes with as open a mind as possible to see things in a new way.

As an example, suppose that a marketing analyst wanted to develop a theory about what motivates people to buy certain items. If the analyst decided to use a theory-generating approach, the research could begin by observing the shopping behavior of people in a mall. The analyst would probably already have some belief, based on theories of behavior and marketing, that advertising does affect behavior. The analyst's perceptions during the observation would not be really pure but would be influenced by theoretic notions about how people shop. However, if the intent of the theory builder is to try to discover some previously unaccounted for variable or to describe something about shopping behavior that has not been described, preconceived ideas about this behavior must be recognized and set as far aside as possible.

One approach to theory-generating research that has been used in nursing is grounded theory (Glaser and Strauss, 1967). This form of field methodology requires the simultaneous processes of collecting, coding, and categorizing empiric observations and forming concepts and relationships based on the data obtained. Grounded-theory methodologies also use deductive approaches to examine propositions of theory. However, it is initially an inductive method.

Other forms of theory-generating research include field observations, as used in anthropology, and participant observation, as used in sociology. The investigator attempts to minimize any intrusion or effect on events observed and seeks to view and describe things occurring as they would if the observer were not present. The investigator attends to clues about how one event affects another and explains the things observed by developing theoretic relationship statements about those observations (Stern, 1980).

Because many phenomena cannot be observed directly, theory-generating research must sometimes use indirect ways of gathering data. Phenomenology is one example of this approach. Phenomenology as a research method is designed to describe the subjective, lived experiences of people and to comprehend the meanings that people place on these experiences (Benner, 1994). These experiences cannot be observed; they are directly accessible only to the person who has the experience. Indirect ways of observing empiric reality include interviewing or questioning individuals about what they feel or remember or how they respond to certain situations. Feelings, thoughts, memories, dreams, and private human experiences can be observed only through how people choose to relate them.

Different inductive methodologies produce different types of knowledge and different forms of descriptive statements or theories. Grounded-theory methods result in relationship statements or propositions that the researcher has observed in empiric experiences. Phenomenology results in interpretive narratives that describe meaning as fully as possible. Regardless of the approach, inductive investigators whose purpose is to contribute empiric knowledge for the discipline address issues of soundness by systematically organizing and describing their research results.

Theory-Validating Research

Once theory is constructed, by whatever means, it is possible to use research methods for validation. The methods are designed to ascertain how accurately the theory depicts phenomena and their relationships. Theoretic statements can be translated into questions and hypotheses so long as the abstractions of the theory can be directly or indirectly represented with empiric indicators. A single study is usually based on one or two relational statements from among several that might possibly be extracted from a theory. No one study can test the entirety of a theory. Some theories contain some relationship statements that can be tested and other relationship statements that cannot be tested by research because empiric indicators cannot be identified.

Even though a theory has been incompletely tested, it is regarded as relatively sound if several research studies conducted over time in different settings demonstrate a degree of confidence in the theory. If some statements are supported by research, whereas others are unsupported or refuted by research, the research provides a basis for revising the theory or developing new theory.

Theory-validating research is usually thought of as a deductive approach. The research starts with an abstract relational statement derived from theory. From the theoretic statement, hypotheses or research questions are created for a specific research situation.

Research questions may also be used in theory-validating research. This type of research typically uses descriptive and correctional designs. The concepts in the research questions are empirically represented, and observations are made. The data are collated and described in such a way that the questions are addressed and implications related to the development of the theory are stated.

Because hypotheses must contain a relationship between at least two variables, the research design is usually an experimental, quasi-experimental, or correlational approach (Polit and Hungler, 1995). In theory-validating research, the investigator deliberately changes or controls conditions so that the study clearly focuses on the nature of the relationship between the variables that have been selected for study. Several descriptive and relationship validating studies are usually needed to validate and extend a theory because only a limited number from among all possible relationships can be included in one study. A single study can contribute appreciably to the validation process if it is theoretically sound.

In the following sections we examine the general research process and identify how both theory-generating and theory-validating research can be designed and therefore evaluated to achieve the most value from the research effort.

DEVELOPING SOUND THEORETIC RESEARCH

The research process can be examined for theoretic soundness at each stage. The following descriptions of each stage can serve as a guide for developing or evaluating the theoretic soundness of a research study. Examples are given in each section from two research studies to illustrate features of theory-validating and theory-generating research. The example of theory-generating research used a grounded-theory approach to generate hypotheses concerning the social process of reimaging that occurs in response to significant alternations in physical appearance or functioning of the body

(Norris, Kunes-Connell, and Spelic, 1998). The example of theory-validating research used a quasi-experimental design to test a middle-range theory of homelessness-helplessness derived from Miller's model of patient power resources (Tollett and Thomas, 1995).

The Clinical Problem, Research Purpose, Research Problem, and Hypotheses

In theory-linked research the purpose, the problem statements, and the hypotheses are designed to show the relationships between the chosen theory base and the particular study being conducted. In theory-validating research, each of these statements should be explicitly formulated because they direct movement from the broad, general intent to the empiric specifics of the study. In descriptive and exploratory theory-validating research, hypotheses may not be stated or labeled as such, and research problems (questions) are developed. Although not necessarily stated in relationship form, the questions imply underlying relationships of significance to the developing theory.

In theory-generating research, only the clinical and research problems are required; the other statements may or may not be developed explicitly in the course of the research process. They are not necessarily explicitly stated in published reports of completed research, but in well-reported studies the statements appropriate to each approach can be inferred from the text of the published article.

In theory-validating research, statements of purpose, problem, and hypotheses or questions are formulated in advance of conducting the data-gathering activity. In theory-generating research, the purpose and problem statements are formulated in advance; if relationships are stated, they are derived from the data. Table 5-1 describes the purpose served by each type of statement and shows how clinical problem, research purpose, research problem, and hypotheses follow from each other and provide a conceptual link between the theory and the research study. As the table shows, there are two types of problems: clinical and research.

The clinical problem is a question that reflects the general experiential concern that generated or influenced the study and suggests the study context. The clinical problem clearly reflects the experiential questions that are fundamental to developing empiric knowledge: What is this? How does it work?

The research purpose indicates whether the study is theory-generating or theory-validating in nature and whether the study focuses on description, explanation, or prediction. If the study is for the purpose of generating theory, the purpose further states the empiric reality the investigator is

TABLE 5-1 Comparison of Clinical Problem, Research Purpose, Research Problem, and Hypothesis Statements in Theory-Linked Research

Type of Statement	What the Statement Conveys	Theory-Generating*	Theory-Validating†
Clinical problem	Specifies the experiential observations that generated or influenced the study	How do people recover following a disruption in body image?	What can be done to instill hope in homeless people to enable them to move on with the process of re-establishing themselves in society?
Research purpose	Specifies whether the research is theory generating or theory validating	To generate a grounded theory of adaptation to body image disruption over the 18-month period following an alteration in physical appearance or function	To test a midrange theory of the homelessness-hopelessness cycle with a nursing intervention designed to instill hope in homeless persons
Research problem	Poses a question to be answered Is less general than the purpose and makes clear how the purpose is to be achieved Expresses the nature of the variable or events to be studied Implies the empiric possibilities for the abstract concepts given in the purpose Expresses the relationships between concepts if the relationship is the focus for the study	What are the perceptions and experiences of people in recovery after an alteration in physical appearance or function?	Does a specific nursing intervention increase hope, self-efficacy, and self-esteem and decrease depression in homeless persons?

*Data from Norris J, Kunes-Connell M, Spelic SS: A grounded theory of reimaging, *Adv Nurs Sci* 20:1, 1998.

†Data from Tollett JH, Thomas SP: A theory-based nursing intervention to instill hope in homeless veterans, *Adv Nurs Sci* 18:76, 1995.

Continued

TABLE 5-1 Comparison of Clinical Problem, Research Purpose, Research Problem, and Hypothesis Statements in Theory-Linked Research—cont'd

Type of Statement	What the Statement Conveys	Theory-Generating*	Theory-Validating†
Hypothesis	Indicates the specific choices made in relation to the variables for the study Implies the design of the study Implies the type of analysis used	*Developed from the findings of the study* Reimaging, the basic social process that occurs in response to significant alterations in physical appearance or functioning of the body, consists of three phases: body image disruption, wishing for restoration, and reimaging the self. Each individual's journey through the reimaging process is facilitated by three action processes: assimilation, accommodation, and interpretation.	*Posed at the outset of the study to guide the research methodology.* There will be higher scores on measures of hope, self-efficacy, and self-esteem and lower scores on a measure of depression in subjects receiving a specific nursing intervention to instill hope than in subjects who receive the usual and customary treatment.

studying. If the study is theory validating, the purpose states the theoretic frame of reference for the study.

For both theory-generating and theory-validating research, the research problem is less general than the statement of purpose and directs the more specific, circumstantial focus of the study. The research problem is phrased in the form of a question that implies how the purpose of the study is to be achieved. It reflects the variables or events to be studied and implies that empiric possibilities for abstract concepts to be developed are embodied in existing theoretic relationships.

When hypotheses are stated, they indicate the circumstantial restrictions of the study, reflect the study design, and suggest the analysis to be made of data. Hypotheses usually provide specific guidance for statistical analysis of quantitative data. If the analysis of the research data does not depend on statistics for drawing conclusions, hypotheses might not be stated; rather, research questions are used to guide data analysis.

In theory-generating research, hypotheses may or may not be stated. Problem statements or research questions may be appropriate for guiding a study intended to generate theory, and hypotheses are formulated at the conclusion of the study, if at all. When formulated, hypotheses provide specific direction for future research.

Background of the Study and Literature Review

In all research, the literature review surveys research findings that are pertinent to the study that is being conducted. In theory-linked research, the literature review also includes a summary evaluation of the theoretic background for the study.

For theory-generating research, the background for the study includes a review of previous work, pertinent to the area of concern. The author's thinking and experience are important as background for the study. The literature review is comprehensive and continues throughout the data-gathering and analysis phases. As the ideas and concepts emerge from the data, the researcher uses the data to guide explorations in the existing literature. The empiric observations remain the primary source for analysis and interpretation, but in some instances the literature provides a basis for refining and delineating central concepts and the relationships between them.

In theory-validating research, previous studies based on the theory form a substantial portion of the literature review. The review also contains a critique of previous research based on alternative theories and on concepts or variables shown to be related to the study's central purpose. The review traces how the study has been conceived and summarizes the theoretic ideas that are being tested. It clarifies how and why specific relationships within the theory are being tested.

In Table 5-1, Tollett and Thomas's theory-validating study (1995) is used to show how statements of clinical problem, research purpose, research problem, and hypotheses are formulated. In this study report the background includes a description of Miller's patient power resources model and Tollett's theory of homelessness-hopelessness derived from Miller's model. The background focuses on explaining the way in which the study variables were conceptualized and the assumptions on which the study was based. The background includes a review of literature related to each of the study variables and the instruments that were selected for measurement of each variable.

Norris, Kunes-Connell, and Spelic's report (1998) illustrates the conception of a research idea from questioning how people adjust after a major alteration in body structure or function. The literature they reviewed revealed that the existing research on body image and self-esteem after body alterations was predominantly quantitative and cross-sectional, focusing on particular body alterations at specific times. From their perspective the existing literature on people's experience of body alteration offered insufficient background for building concepts and theoretic relationships that are needed to understand how people adjust over time to this type of major life-altering event.

The Research Methodology

Several concerns with regard to research method must be carefully considered when theory-linked research is undertaken: the means of obtaining the data, the selection of the sample for study, the design of the research, and the analysis of data and conclusions.

The Means of Obtaining Data. How the data are collected or recorded must be consistent with the purpose of the research design. For theory-generating research, the study is usually descriptive in nature and requires either directly or indirectly observing and recording empiric events that the investigator does not alter during the course of study. Theory-validating research also draws on these means of obtaining data. Because this type of research often relies on some type of experimental or correlational analysis, the tools and assessment guides used tend to be those that yield quantitative measures of the variables.

Direct observation requires being physically present. Data are recorded by some means, such as note taking, audiotaping, or videotaping. Examples include watching and making notations about behavior during the process of mother-infant interactions, about interactions between nurses and clients within an intensive care unit, and about the behavior of a person experiencing a crisis such as pain.

Indirect observation includes the following: interviews; questionnaires and standardized tools that elicit feelings, thoughts, or memories; and self-reports of experiences not directly observable. Tools and assessment guides designed to elicit reports about selected phenomena must be carefully examined to be sure they can provide the evidence needed to achieve the purposes of the study. Tools developed with a particular theoretic bias introduce a perspective that may not be desirable in theory-generating research. In theory-validating research, the means of obtaining data must be carefully considered in relation to the theoretic adequacy of tools and assessment approaches. In both types of research, the problems of reliability and validity of both direct and indirect observations are considered. Tools that are designed to yield a numeric score are assessed for reliability and validity via statistical methods. Interview approaches that are designed to produce narrative descriptions are examined carefully to ascertain how well the approach will function to elicit the type of responses that are needed. The research report should include a discussion of the level of development for the tools used, what theoretic perspective underlies any tools used, and what evidence exists of the tool's reliability and validity.

In Tollett and Thomas's study (1995) the Miller Hope Scale was selected to measure hope because it was developed by the theorist whose ideas guided the study. The other instruments used were evaluated for their theoretic consistency with the perspectives of the study, as well as for their recognized reliability and validity in measuring the constructs they were designed to measure. The scales used were the Self-Efficacy Scale (SES), The Rosenberg Self-Esteem Scale (RES), and the Beck Depression Inventory (BDI).

In Norris, Kunes-Connell, and Spelic's study (1998) of reimaging after body alteration, data were collected by interviews with a broad interview guide. The interview guide focused on participants' perceptions of themselves and their experiences prior to and throughout the study, their thoughts, feelings, adaptive strategies, and perceptions of the responses of others. Participants were interviewed at home or another place of their choice at 3, 6, 12, and 18 months following the physical alteration.

The Selection of the Sample. The selection of the sample is essentially what limits the research to a particular time and place. It is a part of the research that links the abstractions of the theory with empiric phenomena. In theory-generating research, the investigator begins with the following assumption:

> There is some phenomenon or event happening in reality that will be evident if I observe this particular group of people. Furthermore, this particular group is sufficiently like other groups of people who have this experience to represent them.

The individuals chosen for the sample are purposely selected because they can contribute information and insight related to the phenomenon that is being studied.

In theory-validating research, sample selection requires the investigator to take the position that if the theory is empirically reasonable, it will be supported by what happens with the specific persons selected for study, or, if the theory is not empirically accurate, the responses of the sample studied will refute the theory. Because most theory-validating research relies on statistical analysis of quantitative data, sample selection is guided by the requirements of statistical analysis. Both the population to whom the theoretic relationship applies and the sample that is being tested must be specified. Drawing the conclusion of empiric accuracy of the relationship depends on the assumption that the statistical requirements for sampling from the identified population have been met.

In Norris, Kunes-Connell, and Spelic's study (1998) of reimaging after body alteration, participants were contacted by advertisements in newspapers and through health professionals. Purposive sampling was used to ensure a variety of ages and types of physical changes. Twenty-eight individuals, ranging in age from 19 to 85, completed all aspects of the study. Body image disruptions included rapid weight gain or loss in excess of 50 pounds; amputation or paralysis of body parts; scars from burns, surgery, or trauma; ostomies; surgical reconstruction; and cardiac transplantation.

In the report of Tollett and Thomas's theory-validating study (1995), the sample consisted of forty homeless veterans who were assigned randomly to a waiting control group or the treatment group. The waiting control group received the intervention following completion of measurement of the study variables.

The Research Design. The design of the research outlines the procedure and contingencies used for answering the research questions or testing the hypotheses. In theory-generating research, the design must be consistent with the theory-generating orientation of the research. It often involves observation of a particular kind of phenomenon of interest in given groups. Stern (1980) described the design of grounded theory as a matrix in which several research processes are in operation at once. The investigator examines obtained data and begins to code, categorize, conceptualize, and write impressions about its meaning.

Sometimes research designs that are typically used in theory-validating research are needed for theory-generating research. This is the case when a sequence of ordinarily occurring events is an area of concern. For example, suppose something happens to create a sequence of events, such as the birth of a child or the death of a loved one. The research interest might be to describe the usual responses of individuals over a period of time, both before and after this event, to generate theory regarding how people live through these situations. In these instances, comparative assessments over time are needed. The investigator does not, as in classic experimental designs, impose the changes as a part of the design but rather waits for the changes to occur. The investigator then describes the nature of outcomes that occur before and after the event to develop theory.

Theory-generating research also may require comparison groups that are typical of experimental designs in order to determine if a phenomenon occurs only under certain circumstances. Suppose, for example, that an investigator wanted to determine if body image formation is appreciably affected by chronic illness. The phenomenon could be studied by comparing body image formation in a group of people who have a chronic illness with body image formation in a group who do not have chronic illness. The comparison would determine whether aspects of the phenomenon of body image formation are unique to people with chronic illness. This information would contribute to the development of theory related to body image formation.

In some forms of theory-validating research, the researcher deliberately alters circumstances in some way to test the relationships expressed in the hypotheses. The design usually includes some intervention or investigator-created circumstances consistent with the theoretic basis for the study.

In Tollett and Thomas's theory-validating study (1995), a pretest, posttest, quasi-experimental design was used. Each veteran responded to the study instruments at the time of admission to the study, after which for 4 weeks the treatment group participated in 12 60-minute small group sessions led by the nurse researcher. The waiting control group received the usual treatment during this same 4-week period. At the end of the 4 weeks, the participants again completed the study instruments, and the waiting control group received the nursing intervention to instill hope.

Norris, Kunes-Connell, and Spelic's study (1998) of reimaging after body alteration used a grounded-theory design. The grounded-theory approach provides a continuous and interactive process that promotes a fit between what people actually experience and the theory that emerges as a result of coding that experience. As the interviews were transcribed, they were coded, and a constant comparative method was used to identify additional areas for exploration in upcoming interviews.

Analysis of the Data and Conclusions. The analysis of data in theory-linked research must be consistent with the purposes of the research and the research design. For theory-generating research, analysis of data involves narrative, descriptive, and other relatively qualitative types of analysis. Depending on the type of observation used, a quantitative, numeric, or statistical analysis of the data can also be presented, but it is accompanied by a theoretic analysis that includes the full range of observations and the ways in which the observations occurred.

In a grounded-theory approach, analysis of the data involves coding and categorizing the observations. In participant observation, the analysis may report sample observations that typify the characteristic events or the sequence of events that was observed. Whatever the form of data presentation, the investigator proposes concepts generated from the data and, if possible, a description of theoretic propositions that emerge from the data. The extent to which concepts and theoretic propositions are formulated depends on how well the evidence supports making conceptual and theoretic formulations and on the extent to which previous studies support such conceptual and theoretic development.

In theory-validating research, analysis of the data should present sufficient quantitative and qualitative evidence to support or reject the hypotheses or to address the research questions. The conclusions of the study should include an interpretive analysis of the findings in relation to the theory being tested. The analysis of data focuses on the specific study findings, whereas the conclusions focus on the theoretic significance of the study.

In Norris, Kunes-Connell, and Spelic's grounded-theory method (1998), the data analysis involved coding transcriptions from taped interviews and field notes and examining the units of analysis for patterns through the technique of constant comparative analysis. Patterns were then analyzed for new categories and concepts. The relationships among the categories and concepts gave form to the findings of the study. The process of data analysis led to the description of the stages of the process of reimaging and to the identification of action processes that facilitate each individual's journey through the reimaging process (see Table 5-1).

In Tollett and Thomas's theory-validating study (1995), the pretest and posttest scores for both groups were analyzed with an analysis of covariance procedure with pretest scores as the covariate. There was a significant difference between the control and treatment groups in the levels of hope, but no other significant differences were found, even though they all changed in the hypothesized direction. The pretest and posttest scores for the treatment group were examined using paired t tests, showing significant changes in levels of hope, self-esteem, and depression. The control group pretest and posttest scores showed no significant differences on any of the variables. Based on these findings, the authors conclude that the study provides support for the midrange theory of homelessness-hopelessness cycle.

Generalizability and Usefulness of the Study

In theory-linked research, one of the important considerations for a single study is how it contributes to theory development. In most instances, a single study raises more questions than it answers, and questions raised must be presented to provide a basis for future study. Theory-generating research should result in relationship statements that can be studied and used in further developing the theory. Theory-validating research may result in evidence that suggests revision or extension of the theory tested, or it may suggest an entirely new avenue for development of theory.

Theory-generating research is often immediately useful for practice because of its grounding in the experience for which the theory is designed. Theory-generating research often also provides a basis for further theory-related work based on new insights and new questions. Theory-validating research can also have immediate practice application. If the research design is valid and the findings are generalizable and consistent with related research findings, the investigator may conclude that certain approaches in the realm of practice might be useful. However, immediate use in practice cannot always be expected. The primary value of theory-validating research is to stimulate further study and theory development that will add to empiric knowledge on which practice can be based.

CONCLUSION

To develop sound theory in nursing, empiric methods are used to refine concepts and theoretic relationships. Research approaches begin with such questions as What is it? and How does it work? Research methods can be used to generate theory or to replicate or validate the adequacy of existing theory. In the next chapter we examine approaches to replication and validation of empiric knowledge in practice.

Reference List

Benner P: The tradition and skill of interpretive phenomenology in studying health, illness, and caring practices. In P Benner, editor: *Interpretive phenomenology: embodiment, caring and ethics in health and illness,* Thousand Oaks, Calif, 1994, Sage.

Bleich D: *Subjective criticism,* Baltimore, 1978, Johns Hopkins University Press.

Dubin R: *Theory building,* rev ed, New York, 1978, Free Press.

Ferrans CE: Development of a conceptual model of quality of life. In Gift AG, editor: *Clarifying concepts in nursing research,* New York, 1997, Springer.

Ferrans CE, Powers M: Psychometric assessment of the quality of life index, *Res Nurs Health* 15:29, 1992.

Glaser B, Strauss A: *The discovery of grounded theory,* Chicago, 1967, Aldine.

Greer S: *The logic of social inquiry,* Chicago, 1969, Aldine.

Gunter LM: Research techniques applied to nursing, *Nurs Res* 13:230, 1964.

Lincoln YS, Guba EG: *Naturalistic inquiry,* Newbury Park, Calif, 1985, Sage.

Newman MA: *Theory development in nursing,* Philadelphia, 1979, FA Davis.

Norris J, Kunes-Connell M, Spelic SS: A grounded theory of reimaging, *Adv Nurs Sci* 20:1, 1998.

Polit B, Hungler B: *Nursing research,* ed 5, Philadelphia, 1995, JB Lippincott.

Reed E: *Sexism and science,* New York, 1978, Pathfinder Press.

Reynolds PD: *A primer in theory construction,* Indianapolis, 1971, Bobbs-Merrill.

Scheffler I: *Science and subjectivity,* Indianapolis, 1967, Bobbs-Merrill.

Silva MC, Rothbart D: An analysis of changing trends in philosophies of science on nursing theory development and testing, *Adv Nurs Sci* 6:1, 1984.

Stern PN: Grounded theory methodology: its uses and processes, *Image J Nurs Sch* 12:20, 1980.

Tollett JH, Thomas SP: A theory-based nursing intervention to instill hope in homeless veterans, *Adv Nurs Sci* 18:76, 1995.

Chapter 6

Replicating and Validating Empiric Knowledge in Practice

Practice is goal directed. Clinical testing of theory is therefore essential.
Choose your theory—it does not hold in all circumstances. The
professional must not be just a simple user of theory, but a developer,
a tester and expander of theory. Not for the purpose of scholarship,
but for intelligent practice.

Rosemary Ellis (1969, p. 1435)

Development of empiric knowledge, such as theories and models for a practice discipline, requires the processes of replication and validation in the practice setting to assess the value of theoretic knowledge for moving toward valued nursing goals. Research methods are used in these processes, and the findings contribute to the development of the theory being applied. Practice-based replication and validation of theory contribute to the development of scientific competence among nurses and, in turn, contribute to improving the quality of nursing care. We use the phrase "deliberative application and validation" to refer to the use of empiric knowledge to guide practice and to practice-oriented approaches that contribute to empiric knowledge development. Deliberative application and validation of theory involve the use of practice to (1) refine conceptual meaning and (2) validate theoretic relationships and outcomes in practice.

By practice, we mean the experiences a nurse encounters during the process of caring for people. Some experiences are those of the client, others are those of the nurse, some are interactive, and some are environmental. These experiences occur in many settings, but, when they occur in the context of providing nursing care, they are considered part of nursing practice.

In this chapter we address specific ways in which practitioners contribute to empiric knowledge development processes and ways in which empiric knowledge development processes contribute to practice. We discuss important dimensions of refining conceptual meaning that can be accomplished only in the context of practice, and present guidelines for validating theoretic relationships and outcomes of practice and guidelines for methodologic approaches to validating theoretic relationships and outcomes.

REFINING CONCEPTUAL MEANING

The perceptual experiences from which nursing concepts develop are found in the practice of nursing. Practicing nurses who reflect on the nature of their experiences and systematically communicate their reflections make significant contributions to replicating and validating empiric knowledge. Individuals who are primarily involved in knowledge development benefit from the ideas of many nurses who practice nursing. Individuals do not participate equally in all processes required for the development of empiric knowledge; rather, individual nurses participate in a collective endeavor.

Empiric concepts are formed from nursing practice by observing, naming, and making sense of what happens. The processes we describe in Chapter 3 for creating conceptual meaning can be used to systematically document your reflections concerning your experiences, from which you can derive a tentative conclusion about the experience you particularly want to study. Because your thinking will be grounded in your nursing practice, you have a rich resource from which to explore conceptual meanings. Once you have tentatively described your phenomenon of interest, you can turn to activities for refining conceptual meaning. There are four practice-dependent activities required for refining conceptual meaning.

Identifying Empiric Indicators

Practice provides essential evidence that is used to select empiric indicators for abstract concepts. The experiences of practice can challenge existing theoretic conceptualizations, and they can reveal hunches that have not yet been linked to a particular concept or theory. The basic question is, What have I experienced that can be linked to the abstract concept X?

Anxiety is a good example of such an experience. Suppose that a wide range of behaviors observed in practice are described in a theory as manifestations of the concept of anxiety. These behaviors might include wringing of hands, silence and refusing to talk, excessive talking, laughing, crying, sweating, compulsive eating, or not eating (lack of appetite). Tools have been constructed that assess the concept by using these empiric indicators. In your practice experience you observe that these ideas do not always fit. When you work with individuals who are anxious, you observe that they tend to behave in ways that are not consistent with the theoretic concept. There are some behaviors that you almost never observe; others that are commonly experienced are not taken into account by the theory. Because anxiety as an abstract idea does convey something that you know exists, it might be helpful if you could better identify it, understand how it works, and determine how people experience it differently. As you draw on your experience, new ideas begin to emerge from the empiric behaviors you have noticed.

Differentiating Similar Concepts

Concepts that are similar yet different might share certain empiric indicators, and differentiating them may be difficult. If knowing the difference between them is important in practice, practice can provide the empiric information and conceptual insights required to distinguish them. This purpose becomes critical when you realize that errors can be made in assigning meaning to a person's experience. For example, you might have been taught that certain behaviors are manifestations of anxiety, based on a popular theory of anxiety. You have developed an approach to help anxious people reduce their anxiety and improve their function, but it does not seem to be as effective as you think it should be. One problem might be that the behaviors are not indicative of anxiety but are associated with fear. Your challenge is to begin to conceptualize anxiety more clearly, conceptualize what else might be happening, and begin to find ways to differentiate between the experiences of anxiety and fear. As you question and challenge the conceptualization and the conclusions that you draw from it, you will form a basis for restructuring the concepts and form new or revised concepts that better represent nursing experience.

Identifying New Concepts

Creating conceptual meaning is a process that can lead to identification of new concepts. Model, borderline, related, and contrary cases that come from practice reflect the richness and complexity of practice. As you reflect deliberatively on these situations, your insights can lead to new ideas that contribute to forming new concepts.

For example, suppose you begin to notice that something about how people learn in the postoperative period does not seem to be described in any of the literature you have read. Most learning theories have been developed and tested within classroom or laboratory settings, where learners are students or other types of healthy subjects. In nursing situations, the learner is often experiencing an altered health state, and the patterns of behavior that are the focus of learning in this context have not been addressed in developing concepts and theories of learning. As you reflect on your experience, you see meanings that are different from the meaning of learning in the existing learning theories. As you discuss your ideas with other nurses, you find that they have made similar observations. From this awareness, you can build a new conceptualization that, once named, can be incorporated into theory and used in practice.

Identifying Conceptual and Diagnostic Criteria

Although criteria for nursing diagnoses are not the same as criteria for a concept in theory development, nursing diagnostic criteria can be derived partially from criteria for a concept, and vice versa. Nursing diagnostic criteria take into account generally accepted standards for practice, as well as knowledge and application of many areas of theory that are pertinent to the diagnosis. Consider, for example, the nursing diagnosis "altered parenting related to inappropriate and/or non-nurturing parenting behaviors as evidenced by impaired parental-infant attachment." In practice, the purpose is to accurately identify this problem in order to provide effective nursing care. The phrase "altered parenting related to inappropriate and/or non-nurturing parenting behaviors" implies knowledge of how certain behaviors affect parental-infant attachment. The phrase "impaired parental-infant attachment" implies knowledge of human attachment theory and also suggests the focus for nursing actions. When criteria for nursing diagnoses are derived in part from a concept not yet well developed, the process of creating conceptual meaning can be used to form tentative diagnostic criteria that can be tested for empiric accuracy or validity.

The criteria for the nursing diagnosis of "altered parenting related to inappropriate and/or non-nurturing parenting behaviors" could include conceptual criteria for parenting. The diagnostic criteria also include value qualifiers, such as the term *altered*, that convey the value that the practitioner assigns to a situation in the process of making clinical decisions. When the parent under consideration is the mother, the diagnostic criteria might be as follows:

- Visual contact between mother and infant is minimal or absent.
- Physical touching of the infant by the mother is limited to necessary touch.

- There is minimal or no vocalization directed by mother to infant.
- The mother's verbal expressions focus on herself (that is, concerns for her own body or image or relationships with peers, rather than expressions focusing on the infant).
- Care of the infant is easily or passively given over to another caretaker.

These diagnostic criteria reflect but do not include all conceptual criteria for mothering we gave as an example in Chapter 3, which were as follows:

- Visual contact must be observed to be directed from the mothering person to the person who receives mothering.
- The person who receives mothering must be physically touched by the mothering person.
- Some positive feeling must be experienced by the mothering person and by the person who receives mothering.
- There must be a reciprocal interaction between the mothering person and the person who receives mothering.
- Vocalization by the mothering person must occur.

Notice that the diagnostic criteria specify an altered interaction, whereas the conceptual criteria point to observations that signify "mothering." The diagnostic criteria focus on those aspects that are relatively accessible to being empirically observed and assessed in practice. The conceptual idea of "some positive feeling" could potentially be operationalized and measured or otherwise assessed, but the many challenges in attempting to do so may not warrant pursuit of this line of development, particularly when more readily accessible indicators, such as visual contact and touch, are suggested and may be adequate for your purpose.

The diagnostic criteria may be adequate for creating standard approaches to practice and may be sufficient to use in formal testing of the theoretic concept. Evidence of the diagnostic criteria recorded in practice provides a basis for decisions about the adequacy of the criteria for either research or practice, as well as direction as to how research should proceed. If the purpose of creating conceptual meaning is to form criteria useful for nursing diagnosis, then traits that are observed in practice and that can be verified and assessed need to be emphasized.

VALIDATING THEORETIC RELATIONSHIPS AND OUTCOMES OF PRACTICE

Deliberatively applying theory involves using research methods to demonstrate how a theory affects nursing practice. It involves processes that place a selected theory within the context of practice to ensure that it serves the goals of the profession. Deliberative validation provides evidence of the theory's usefulness in developing nurses' scientific competence and in ensuring quality of care.

The essence of the theory-practice relationship is deliberatively applying and validating theory. Theory that addresses goals of practice provides a way to systematically develop substantial empiric knowledge within the discipline. Theory is not a quick-and-easy answer to a problem but rather provides knowledge and understanding to ultimately enhance the practice of nursing.

A first step is to ascertain if the theory can be used in practice. Some theories that hold promise may not be sufficiently developed to justify their application. Others might be poorly suited to a particular practice area. The guidelines we suggest in the following section can be used to make this decision. Once you decide to use the theory in practice, you can then design research methods to demonstrate how well the theory contributes to your practice goals through the deliberative validation of theory.

How to Determine If a Theory Should Be Applied and Validated in Practice

Theory ideally serves to improve nursing practice. Usually this goal is achieved by using theory or portions of theory to guide practice. Because theory can be used prematurely or inappropriately, it is important to consider how sound judgments are made regarding the validation of theory in practice.

Even though theory is often seen as not relevant to nursing practice, empiric knowledge is considered to be the foundation for the nursing process in the form of the scientific rationale for nursing care. In practice, judgments are often made without conscious effort or explicit explanation of the basis for the judgment. If called on to do so, most nurses can cite some valid empiric reasons for their judgments. Many common practices in nursing have emerged from sound principles or standards based in fundamental truths that have not yet come under sufficient challenge to be a focus for knowledge development. As Beckstrand (1980) has noted, "Principles of practice are shorthand ways of referring to fundamental truths to be considered and general customs to be followed" (p. 73). Standards of practice reflect valued actions that are generally accepted in a given situation. Principles and standards are judged by their consistent outcomes; for example, do they consistently yield desired results in practice? They are changed not by systematically challenging the standards or the principles themselves but rather by discovering another approach that better achieves the desired outcome (Beckstrand, 1980). Although facts, theories, or models cited as the basis of care may provide explanations that seem rational and well founded, it is important to consider how adequate the ideas are as a basis for making judgments and for directing nursing actions.

Theory cannot be assumed to predict a desired outcome and does not exist to give specific guidelines for what should be done in a given situation. Rather, theory explains possible relationships that can be questioned. The goal of a theory and goals of practice should be consistent, but this cannot be assumed to be the case. If the relationships predicted by a theory are inadequate or do not accurately represent reality, the theory may not be effective in achieving practice goals. Theory can be effectively used to describe, explain, and predict a phenomenon that occurs in practice but may not adequately contribute to the goals of practice if it is applied. Because any application of theory will affect practice, deliberative use of theory cannot be undertaken lightly. The questions we suggest in the following section can be used to reach an informed decision about the use of the theory so that its practice value can be assessed.

Are the Theory Goals and Practice Goals Congruent? To answer this question, examine the goal of the theory and compare it with the outcomes or goals that you see as valuable for nursing practice. The existing standards of practice can be used as one basis for clarifying the values on which your practice is based and the overall goals that your practice should be reflecting. Another basis for identifying practice goals is your own view of nursing and that of nurses with whom you work. If a theoretic goal would lead to a situation that is not congruent with your idea of optimal health, for example, you may not want to use the theory. Sometimes this judgment is not easy and requires deliberate philosophic assumptions about nursing, health, the individual, the environment, and society. For example, application of a theory may be undertaken to determine if the theoretic goal is consistent with the goal of optimal health. If the theoretic goal is adaptation and you are uncertain if this concept is consistent with your idea of optimal health, you could design a trial that uses the theory in practice, observe the outcomes, and then evaluate the consistency of the outcomes in light of your practice goals.

Is the Intended Context of the Theory Congruent with the Practice Situation? This question addresses how well suited the theory is for your situation, given the general ideas of context that are stated or implied theoretically. A theory of pain alleviation, for example, may explain the processes involved in alleviating pain in any instance in which it occurs. As you become familiar with the theory, you realize that it was developed with reference to mature adults, and you work with children. You and your colleagues would need to explore how well the ideas of the theory might transfer to your own situation before you make a decision to proceed with application of the theory.

Is There, or Might There Be, Similarity between Theory Variables and Practice Variables? This question compares the important theoretic variables, expressed as concepts in the theory, with the variables recognized to be directly influencing the practice situation. In some instances important practice variables may not be included in the theoretic relationship statements. For example, a learning theory may not consider the health status of the learner, and the learner is assumed to be a healthy individual. If practice variables are not accounted for in the theory or if there are substantial differences between the theoretic variables and the practice variables, the theory should be applied with caution, if at all. If the theory appears to have value and satisfies the considerations of most people who will be involved in the deliberative validation process, it might be applied with systematic observation of the effect on outcomes, considering the differing variables that occur in practice. Given your observations, you may have a basis to propose revision of the theory to include important practice variables.

Are the Explanations of the Theory Sufficient to Be Used as a Basis for Nursing Action? Responses to this question must be based on expert judgment about the particular nursing actions that are implied within the theory. As an expert nurse, you may find it difficult to describe the basis on which you would judge a theory to be sufficient or not sufficient. One specific approach in forming your ideas is to examine the correspondence between theoretic and practice variables. If variables in the nursing situation are similar to those that are suggested in the theory, you can then consider the nature of the relationships between the concepts of the theory. Examine the extent to which the explanation makes sense in light of your practice. You may feel guarded about the sense of the theory for practice, but you can see that the perspective of the theory is reasonable. In this case, the theory is probably sufficient as a basis for nursing action, but your tentativeness about it leads you to be cautious as you proceed to use it and to plan careful documentation of the relationships you observe in practice.

An example of a sufficient theoretic explanation for application in practice is the mother-infant attachment theory. Hospitalization of children creates a classic separation response in those children who are separated from a significant parent. The theory describes behaviors (variables) that are clearly observed in hospitalized children. The theory also provides explanations for this phenomenon and predictions about the effects of severe or prolonged separation. Moreover, predictions are made concerning healthy outcomes that could be expected if the separation was less intense or more prolonged. The theory provides direction for the nursing actions that are needed. These are not exact actions or specific rules or principles, but the theory does suggest types of actions that reduce separation and promote attachment.

Is There Research Evidence Supporting the Theory? One very influential source of information for deciding whether a theory can be used in practice is research evidence. Sometimes a theorist, in presenting the theory, provides research evidence to support the initial theoretic formulation. If the evidence is convincing and attracts sufficient attention in the discipline, the professional literature will report research that either validates the initial theoretic relationships or does not support the theory. Research reports often suggest limits on the range of applicability of the theory or flaws in the initial theoretic construction, based on the research evidence generated.

Because theories are not unequivocally supported by research evidence, practitioners have the responsibility to determine if the evidence is sufficient to justify application of the theory in practice. This judgment is best made on the basis of several research studies. If there is little or no research evidence to justify application in practice but most of the other concerns have been satisfied, you can feel reasonably comfortable about applying the theory. In this case give particular attention to observing and recording relevant information regarding corresponding theoretic and situational variables and the limits and outcomes of the theory's use in practice.

How Will the Use of This Theory Influence the Practical Function of the Nursing Unit? Before using a theory in practice, you need to consider the ways in which this approach will affect the functioning of the nursing unit and assess the potential for observing and recording factors that are relevant to the theory's application. Successful application will depend on planning for the changes that are required, including the changes that will be needed to gather the research data for deliberative application. Questions to be addressed in planning for application include the following:

- Do nursing personnel need to be oriented to the theory and its application?
- Does the approach require adjustments in the function or processes of the nursing unit?
- Does the approach require additional time or an adjustment in the allocation of time?

- Will the approach require new equipment or other material resources?
- What practical arrangements and materials are needed to enhance the ease and accuracy of making and recording observations?
- How will trial application affect other activities in the setting?
- Are special provisions needed for gathering and storing information?
- How will clients be informed of the approaches that will be used?
- How will the data that are obtained be assessed and analyzed?
- If the theoretic goal is attained or not attained, how will the results be explained or accounted for?
- Have alternative explanations been projected in order to have sufficient information to make a judgment about outcomes?
- How will the results of the experience be compiled to communicate them to others?

If each of these questions can be answered in such a way that application seems feasible and desirable, application is probably indicated.

METHODOLOGIC APPROACHES TO VALIDATION OF RELATIONSHIPS AND OUTCOMES

Methods that are used in the deliberative validation of theory are drawn from evaluation research (Posavac and Carey, 1992; Schroeder and Maibusch, 1984; Smeltzer, Hinshaw, and Feltman, 1987). These methods depend on knowing what outcomes you wish to achieve and on having a well-planned approach for achieving the goal. Evaluation research methods depend on having some means for determining what circumstances exist prior to a deliberative use of a theory or model and on comparing them with the results following the change in practice. Factors associated with the outcomes are usually identified and assessed before beginning and again after the approach has been in place for a specified period of time. The following sections describe quality-related outcomes that you might consider in planning deliberative validation of theoretic relationships.

Expected Outcomes That Flow from Theoretic Reasoning

At the heart of deliberative validation of theory is the idea that the theory suggests goals or outcomes that the profession values, and the fundamental purpose for using the theory is to achieve these goals. The outcomes you identify as flowing from theoretic reasoning are likely to represent a key concept of the theory that requires sound empiric indicators and operational definitions. Your choice of empiric indicators and operational definitions may come from prior research, in which case you need to use the measures and determine their adequacy for your purposes. If existing empiric indicators and operational definitions are not readily available, you will need to invest preliminary time and effort to develop your own.

Scientific Competence of Nurses

Although the primary aim in deliberatively applying theory in practice is improved quality of outcomes for those receiving care, it is also important to verify that nurse scientific competence is enhanced. This "outcome" serves to assure that the positive benefits of applying theory in practice can be sustained over time.

Standards of nursing practice that are accepted by the nursing practice unit can contribute to your choice of ways to assess nurse scientific competence, but because standards of care often reflect minimum acceptable practice, you may consider what extensions of the standards are implied within the theoretic reasoning. For example, a key element of your theory could be specific nursing care actions that signify the concept of "caring," and your standards of care may not reflect or require these actions as part of minimal acceptable practice. In your plan, you will need to integrate empiric indicators for these actions and plan a way to assess these nurse actions as an outcome.

Functional Outcomes

Nursing goals are sometimes defined in terms of how efficiently the work of nursing is done, how cost-effective it is, or how smoothly the work of each individual coordinates with others' work. If these factors have been identified as a problem for a particular unit, the factors that are indicative of the problem need to be clearly specified and assessed prior to applying theory. Once the baseline data are obtained and the approach based on the theory has been in place for a period of time, the measures of functional effectiveness are obtained and compared.

Nurse Satisfaction

Satisfaction with respect to nursing job responsibilities can be closely related to functional outcomes. Nurse job satisfaction can be assessed by such factors as working conditions, relationships with colleagues, personal fulfillment, various types of perceived benefits, and perceived dissatisfactions. A premise underlying the selection of this type of outcome is that if nurses are satisfied with their work situation, the quality of care they provide will improve.

Quality of Care Perceived by Those Who Receive Care

People who receive care can be interviewed to ascertain their perception of the quality of their care. There are several aspects of perceived quality of care that can be assessed, including satisfaction with specific dimensions of care, perceived benefits from the care, and perceived dissatisfactions.

IMPLEMENTING A FORMAL METHOD OF STUDY

The approaches used to deliberatively validate theory in practice can draw on traditional research methods but often shift to include the methods of evaluation and quality-assurance research (Posavac and Carey, 1992). In this type of research, the method is designed to provide evidence of the effect of theoretic knowledge on the overall well-being of people who receive care, on the scientific competence of those who practice nursing, and on the practice setting. Ideally, this type of investigation includes measurement of the key outcomes prior to application of the selected theory in practice in order to demonstrate what changes in practice occur after the theory has been applied.

If, for example, you have a theory of pain alleviation that you wish to validate in practice, you might design a study that would first estimate the quality of nursing care and clients' experiences of pain before the theory is used in practice. Your assessment could include the perspective of nurses, people receiving nursing care, and others involved in caring for people who experience pain. After you have this information, you would begin to use the theory in practice and over time continue to observe the same outcome indicators of quality of care. On the basis of your findings, you could make recommendations for practice and for revisions in the conceptualizations of the theory.

When it is not possible to obtain data before applying the theory, alternative approaches are to obtain population or epidemiologic data related to selected outcomes or to obtain measures from a comparable population or group of people. You then compare your outcomes with the population statistics. This approach is necessary in many types of situations. One such circumstance is nursing care that is directed toward prevention of a negative health experience, such as child abuse. If you have selected a theory that you project will influence the parenting abilities of mothers who are at risk for abusing their children, you are not likely to be able to obtain reliable measures of the outcomes you are seeking to achieve. The mothers you are working with may not have had prior parenting experience, or you may not have been involved in their care before they were identified as high-risk parents. You can obtain population statistics concerning the incidence of child abuse, monitor the incidence of abusive behaviors among the mothers for whom you are providing care, and compare your outcomes with the population statistics. You might also identify a group of mothers who are receiving a different type of care to compare your outcomes with those of a different group.

CONCLUSION

In this chapter we discussed the deliberative application and validation of empiric knowledge in practice, including refining conceptual meaning and validating theoretic relationships and outcomes in practice. We posed questions that you can consider before selecting a theory for replication and validation in practice. An individual nurse or group of nurses can select several options on how they might proceed with any of these activities, depending on the needs of their setting and clients. Having other individuals in the environment who understand and support these activities and who can give information and assistance is a tremendous asset. Nurses who deliberatively attempt to use theory in practice contribute to the scientific competence of nurses and to the disciplinary processes of replication and validation.

Reference List

Beckstrand JA: A critique of several conceptions of practice theory in nursing, *Res Nurs Health* 3:69, 1980.

Ellis R: The practitioner as theorist, *Am J Nurs* 69:1434, 1969.

Posavac EJ, Carey RG: *Program evaluation: methods and case studies,* ed 4, Englewood Cliffs, NJ, 1992, Prentice Hall.

Schroeder PC, Maibusch RM: *Nursing quality assurance,* Rockville, Md, 1984, Aspen.

Smeltzer C, Hinshaw A, Feltman B: The benefits of staff nurse involvement in monitoring the quality of patient care, *J Nurs Quality Assurance* 1:1, 1987.

Chapter 7

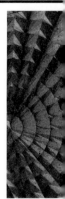

Ethical Knowledge Development

Certain fundamental ethical principles are universal and unchangeable,
but the interpretation and application of truth changes and different
people arrive at truth by widely different methods. . . . Adults who are
dominated by the opinions of the herd may be morally retarded.
We do not act morally unless we act from a sense of conviction
and reason, guided by our own conscience.

Isabel Stewart (1922, pp. 906, 909)

In this chapter we focus on methods for creating ethical knowledge. Figure 7-1 shows the quadrant of our model pertaining to the development of this pattern of nursing knowledge. The figure highlights the creative processes of valuing and clarifying as central for the generation of ethical knowledge forms for nursing, shown in Figure 7-1 as principles and codes. Other forms of ethical knowledge are possible—for example, ethical theories—but we have chosen the forms shown on the model for their central importance to practice.

Like the other patterns, ethical knowledge development begins with ethical knowing. Nurses, regardless of setting, bring to practice the heritage of their own moral development. With this background, nurses reflect on their practice and begin to ask, Is this right? Is this responsible? These questions set into motion the processes of valuing and clarifying. As these questions are answered, knowledge that can be shared is developed.

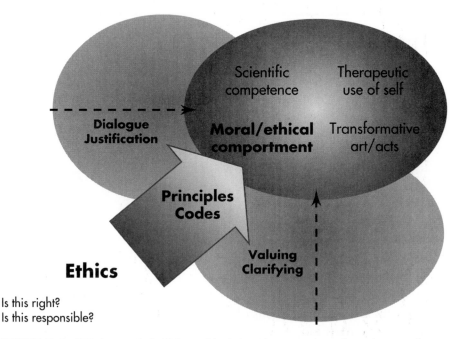

FIGURE 7-1 Valuing and clarifying ethical situations to create formal expressions of ethical knowledge that provide a foundation for moral-ethical comportment.

Through the collective disciplinary processes of dialogue and justification, ethical knowledge is evaluated and understood in relation to practice.

According to our model, nurses who practice using ethical knowledge that has been strengthened through disciplinary processes of dialogue and justification can be expected to increasingly practice with moral-ethical comportment. Moral-ethical comportment, expressed in practice as integrated knowing, can undergo further questioning: Is this right? Is this responsible? As this occurs, the stage is set for the ongoing processes of valuing and clarifying.

In this chapter we begin with a discussion about the nature of ethical and moral knowledge in nursing. Then we consider the processes and forms of ethical knowledge development in nursing that are shown on the model.

ETHICS, MORALITY, AND NURSING

Clearly nursing is a profession that requires ethical knowledge to guide practice. Whether a seasoned nurse or a beginning student, whether working in a high-tech intensive care environment or in a rural, isolated elementary school, the outcomes depend on the nurse's ethical knowing and morality. According to Levine (1989), all nursing actions are moral statements. We would add that all nursing actions are also ethical statements.

Ethics and morality are frequently interchanged and used synonymously in the nursing literature. We see ethics and morality as meshed and use both terms together in this chapter and elsewhere in this book. The distinction between ethics and morality reflects the tension between epistemology and ontology and the difficulty of separating what we know from who we are.

In general, ethics relates to matters of epistemology, whereas morality focuses on ontology. Ethics is a discipline, a branch of inquiry that tries to make sense of what is right or wrong. Ethics, then, is more like head work, the products of which are such things as ethical theories, principles, rules, codes, laws, and lists of obligations or duties and descriptions of ethical-moral behavior. There are two branches of ethics: descriptive and prescriptive. Descriptive ethics is an empiric endeavor that systematizes what people believe ethically and how they behave in relation to those beliefs. For example, suppose you conducted a mall survey and asked passersby (1) if they thought it was wrong to take office supplies to their homes for personal use and (2) if they had ever done this. Collating and reporting their answers would be in the realm of descriptive ethics. Prescriptive or normative ethics is concerned with the "oughts" of behavior. Using cognitive reasoning processes that incorporate emotional and other nonrational sources of behavior, prescriptions for ethical behavior are put into language and set forth as codes, duties, principles, and so forth. Using the mall survey example, you might reason how and why it is not permissible to take office supplies for personal use by invoking a rule that stealing is wrong, and you might then subsequently develop a code of office behavior. In our example, then, the use of descriptive ethics (what is, with regard to beliefs and actions) would reveal that prescriptions for ethical behavior (what ought to be, according to reasoning and logic) are being violated. In this text our focus is on prescriptive ethics, but it is important to recognize the value of descriptive ethics for examining the nature of ethical knowledge in nursing.

Morality, by contrast, is expressed in behavior and grounded in values. If ethics is head work, you might think of morality as heart work. Morality refers to our day-to-day living expressions of what we believe to be good, beliefs that are firmly embedded in culture and in character. When people consistently behave in concert with their values, moral integrity is shown. When moral behavior is blocked by situational factors, moral distress results. Morality is largely determined by culture. People sometimes appeal to some ethical theory or code to justify their actions. More often, morality is shown on a less deliberative and conscious level. Daily expressions of belief about the right, the good, and the noble are filtered through lenses that are influenced by family, friends, religion, gender, and developmental stage. What constitutes moral behavior can thus vary widely, and what is important in one culture (e.g., independence) may be unimportant in another. A religious affiliation associated with one culture may provide a lens that justifies war; another culturally grounded affiliation may offer a lens that justifies pacifism.

Morality and ethics interrelate in that ethical knowledge can provide a template for judging and evaluating moral standards and behavior. The converse is also true, and morality can provide a template for judging ethical knowledge. Ethical principles can be used to challenge morality by providing a system for examining behavior, or ethical knowledge might providing a justification for continuing certain behavior or supporting a particular course of action. Suppose, for example, you felt justified in providing information to a client about alternative health care practices when you knew the primary physician had discouraged the client from using them. Both you and the physician felt your respective actions were moral. Ethical precepts around a client's right to information might be used to justify your action and change the physician's view; ethical precepts relating to protection of the vulnerable might support the physician's view and ultimately change your behavior.

When moral positions collide and both parties hold strong beliefs about their respective positions, there may be no clear answers about how to proceed. In these situations it becomes important to identify the political processes that are operating. If the client's welfare is the concern for both parties, then the nurse should be successful in engaging the physician in dialogue that questions how right and responsible the decision is. Through this process both physician and nurse (and perhaps client) can come to more fully understand the nature of the decision to be made and its potential outcomes. If the physician's attitude reflects more of a power-over, controlling, or paternalistic position in relation to the client, other strategies may be warranted. In this instance the nurse should recognize the nature of power imbalances and how they are sustained and seek avenues that will fundamentally undermine or circumvent the physician's control.

Legal requirements may create moral distress and ethical conflict. Although appeals to ethical knowledge can be used to challenge and justify morality, they do not supersede the law. For example, if you have a strong moral disposition toward counseling an underage woman about her options for birth control but such information is prohibited by state statute, an appeal to ethical knowledge, such as a code of rights, will not get you off the hook in a court of law. In these instances working with professional organizations and within local political circles to change oppressive laws may be warranted. What is important here is to understand that you, as a nurse, may act morally in relation to strong ethical precepts and end up in a court of law because your actions were illegal. Such a risk should be taken knowingly.

Ideally, then, a "good" morality for nursing needs to be in place, with ethical knowledge that supports and justifies yet challenges that morality. Final moral and ethical coherence should be supported by laws and other societal contexts that do not prohibit but allow for its expression.

A quick reference to Figure 7-1 reveals elements of both morality and ethics embedded within the ethical pattern. We have retained the pattern name, ethics, after Carper's (1978) original terminology because our primary focus is on knowledge development, or the ethics of nursing. In this pattern the expressions of ethical knowledge are principles and codes, which reflect the normative or prescriptive focus of ethics. These represent and include the head work of nurses who develop ethical knowledge. The processes whereby such knowledge generates and regenerates involve examining the behavior and claims of nurses—the examination of individual and collective morality.

OVERVIEW OF ETHICAL PERSPECTIVES

Within philosophic ethics various theoretic perspectives have emerged that attempt to set forth the foundation on which to base ethical action. These approaches to ethics have been important for nursing as it attempts to create an ethical perspective on practice. Four perspectives that appear commonly in nursing literature are briefly examined here: relativism, teleology, deontology, and virtue ethics.

Relativism

Relativism is the claim that what constitutes moral action cannot be proven and that the realm of morality and ethics is not an appropriate subject for cognitive reflection. For relativists, ethical systems and morality depend on historical timing, the culture within which the system is embedded, and the particular group within the culture involved in the decision making. Relativism may be a comfortable position to take because it circumvents a responsibility to know how to behave in the face of moral and ethical dilemmas. Under the extreme relativist view, incorporating an idea of moral-ethical comportment into a knowledge development model becomes something of a nonissue because it would be relative to every situation and could not be envisioned as a way to be that would include nurses in general.

Then again, some dimensions of relativism are useful and seem necessary in that nurses often face tremendous clinical complexities in ethical decision making that belie knowing with much certainty what the best course of action is. Despite the fact that moral-ethical decision making involves uncertainties for action that cannot be solved by apriori knowledge of what is moral-ethical, we believe we can move toward a shared idea of what constitutes moral-ethical comportment for nursing.

Teleology and Deontology

Teleology and deontology are two other common labels that reference ethical systems. Most theorylike systems of ethical reasoning or decision making can be broadly classified into one of these two types. In teleology what is right is, or produces, good. Teleologic systems look toward the ends produced by a course of action as the measure to determine the action's goodness. What is a right course of action yields, as expressed in the familiar phrase, the greatest good for the greatest number of people. Taken to extremes, teleologic systems could be used to justify behavior very harmful to a societal group if the harm done produced good for the rest of society. Using teleology one could justify stripping a very wealthy patient of all personal assets for redistribution to the poorer patients and thereby producing a greater good for greater numbers of people.

In deontology what is right may not necessarily be good; that is, deontologic systems separate good from right. A good action may have a bad outcome, as expressed in the phrase the end does not justify the means. In deontologic systems such knowledge forms as external rules or codes determine what is right, regardless of the outcome produced. An extreme view of deontology is exemplified by someone who, required by rule or precept to tell the truth, does so, causing great emotional distress to a client and family. Both deontologic and teleologic systems focus on the individual as a decision maker who is autonomous in action. How the social context imparts meaning and how emotional content and other nonrational forms of behavior affect decision making are not formally considered.

Our system for knowledge development includes aspects of both teleologic and deontologic perspectives. Although the knowledge forms include principles and codes, they are not taken to be infallible or to be followed at all costs. Processes of valuing and clarifying can help elucidate the situational contexts that are important considerations for modification of principles and codes. The disciplinary processes of dialogue and justification can function to temper rules and precepts and sensitize them for different contexts. Also, as the nurse acts, moral-ethical knowledge is integrated with the other knowing patterns to create the best possible ethical-moral decision. This can, in turn, be further examined by questioning, rather than assuming, the rightness and responsibleness of the action.

Virtue Ethics

Virtue ethics introduces the character of the person as an important determiner of moral-ethical decision making. As noted earlier, virtue is unimportant within the frame of reference provided by deontology and teleology. If ethical behavior can be reduced to application of rules or calculations of good, then character would be irrelevant. Character, however, determines how we perceive or frame situations, so a focus on the virtues of the nurse is critically important. Virtue ethics also offers a structure for ethical-moral comportment in the face of relativism by suggesting that a virtuous person will behave in a moral-ethical way. Virtue ethics allows a flexibility in approaching moral-ethical situations that deontologic and teleologic systems do not offer.

However, virtue ethics can be particularly dangerous ethical system for a profession that is gendered in traditional female roles. Some focus on the cultivation of virtuous behavior seems important to ethical knowledge and knowing, but it is important to question who defines what is virtuous and whether an appeal to what the virtuous person would do might be an appeal to what the virtuous (read, submissive, obedient, and self-sacrificing) woman would do. Our model incorporates a focus on virtues through the pattern of personal knowing, but also with regard to processes within the ethical knowledge quadrant. As moral-ethical comportment is integrated with other knowing patterns and then subsequently examined by the questions, Is this right? Is this responsible? we expect that growth toward virtues consistent with praxis will evolve.

NURSING'S FOCUS ON ETHICS AND MORALITY

A focus on the virtues of a dutiful nurse is the focus of much literature on ethics during the first half of the nineteenth century, as noted in Chapter 2. Reverby's (1987) historical work underscores the nature of the nurse's duty to care while denied the means to effect or create an environment where caring was valued and possible.

In more recent nursing literature there has been increasing interest around the concept of caring as a centrally important focus for the development of both empiric and ethical theory. Much of the ethics of care literature centers around the relative merits of an ethic of caring versus an ethic of justice and how moral behavior relates to both.

Nursing's focus on the caring perspective owes much to work that evolved from Carol Gilligan's (1982) critique and challenge of Kohlberg's (1976) theory of moral development. Kohlberg's work staged moral development by using male research subjects, and Gilligan challenged its validity as a normative template for judging moral development in women. Gilligan found that women tended to care about relational concerns that focused on the needs of major players involved in the dilemma. Autonomy in decision making, by contrast, was a central feature of Kohlberg's theory. This theory supported a morality in which actors could remain detached from the situation and appeal to rules as a guide to action. An approach that emphasizes detachment and objectivity in ethical decision making has been linked to traditional medical ethics approaches and critiqued as inappropriate for nursing.

Fry (1989) has suggested that the context of nursing practice requires a moral view of the person rather than a theory of moral action or system of moral justification. For Fry, caring as a moral value ought to be central to any theory of ethics. Others have pointed out that concerns for autonomy and justice that are central to biomedical ethics have been traditionally male-gendered traits. Not only do these imply a separate-from or autonomous stance toward ethical challenges but also they may be inappropriate for nursing, where gendered traits are female (Condon, 1992). Crowley (1994) outlines how Noddings's (1984) ethic of care might be used as a guide to transforming curriculum and subsequently approaches to moral comportment in practice.

Feminists (Hoaglund, 1990; Houston, 1990; Liaschenko, 1993) have criticized the alignment of moral decision making in women with care perspectives because of its potential to further entrench oppressive values. These authors point out the political reality of caring and urge caution lest we embrace a *feminine,* not a *feminist,* ethics (Liaschenko, 1993).

We believe that nurses must be concerned with issues of both care and justice if nursing's purpose is to be realized. As Walker (1993) suggests, nurses' moral expertise is not a question of mastering codes and laws but a matter of being architects of moral space within the health care setting and mediators in the conversations taking place. To do this requires attention to the vulnerabilities of an ethic of care as well as the vulnerabilities of an ethic of justice. As Cooper (1991) puts it, we must take seriously the moral demands of care in the development of ethics. Doing so requires radical responses and moral courage as well as political astuteness. Ethical choices should be guided not only by roles and principles but also by thoughtful analysis of feelings, intuitions, and experiences (Cooper, 1991).

PROCESSES FOR ETHICAL KNOWLEDGE DEVELOPMENT

Our view of ethics is in concert with Carper's original conceptualization of the ethical pattern, which included dimensions of both morality and ethics intersecting with legally prescribed duties. Moreover, no one ethical or moral view is embraced, but there is a constant need to be vigilant about the sociopolitical context within which nurses function.

> The ethical component of nursing is focused on matters of obligation or what ought to be done. Knowledge of morality goes beyond simply knowing the norms or ethical codes of the discipline. It includes all voluntary actions that are deliberate and subject to the judgment of right and wrong. (Carper, 1978, p. 20)

In examining the nature of ethical knowing and knowledge, the questions naturally arise, Toward what end should ethical knowledge be developed? What ought to be done in practice to earn the label *ethical* or *moral?* What values support nursing's ethics and morality? Toward what clinical ends should ethical theories reason and ethical principles move us? What sort of moral development perspective should we embrace and encourage? In the context of teleology we might ask, How do we know what the greatest good is? In the context of deontology, How do we know which rules are good and which are not? For virtue ethics, Which virtues are worthwhile for us to cultivate? Such questions relate to the final value from which no others can be derived, which centers our knowledge development efforts and professional activities. Although we will not answer these questions, we do provide some suggestions toward creating answers. Because our model combines aspects of each of these positions, it is a central question to which we must attend.

As the products and processes within this quadrant of the model are discussed in the next sections, some answers will be provided, but additional questions will be raised. For us the merit of ethical knowledge forms will be judged on the basis of their ability to contribute to praxis. This implies increasing the reflective awareness or consciousness of participants in the practice of nursing. It implies a move toward action grounded in an open awareness and choice for client and nurse—a move toward health. It implies a move to reduce the moral distress nurses face as they encounter and move through ethical and moral dilemmas.

The pattern of ethics as we conceptualize it includes the usual day-to-day, moral decision making that nurses engage in. Ethics goes far beyond what many tend to think of as ethics—the weighty, dramatic decisions often involving end-of-life contexts or controversial political issues. Important ethical knowing is employed and created in everyday incidents. Ethical knowing is reflected in the decision to ignore a comment or attend to it, what to say, what not to say, or whether to keep information to ourselves or reveal it. The ethical decision making that occurs around a conference table, while important, is not our major focus or the major domain of nursing's moral-ethical practice. Rather, ethics as used here concerns everyday uses of morality and ethical knowledge as expressed in ethical comportment in typical practice settings. Nursing's ethics-morality is an everyday ontology.

Ethical knowledge development fundamentally comes from the questioning of moral-ethical comportment—that is, who we are as ethical and moral beings and what we believe is good and right. We assume that nurses bring to their work some base set of values that guide their ethical decisions and moral behavior. As they work within the everyday world, their moral-ethical selves are challenged daily. For example, a nurse might wonder, Should I reveal to an elderly woman that her family is cleaning out her apartment and don't intend to allow her to return home? Should I share my views about what is responsible childbearing for a couple who discover they are both genetic carries for cystic fibrosis? Would this cause more harm than good? What would be gained? For whom? If you reflect for a moment, several instances where you have been faced with such ordinary decisions should come to mind. You will probably notice that your decisions are made relatively quickly without obvious reference to ethical theory, codes, or principles.

The place we begin with discussions of knowledge development for ethics is with the questions, Is [was] this right? Is [was] this responsible? As you work as a nurse, this type of questioning is in the background, for without such questioning you would be unable to make day-to-day moral-ethical moves. This deliberative questioning leads to the creation and re-creation of shared knowledge.

As you or others inquire about the rightness and responsibleness of context-embedded ethical decisions, different perspectives on the decision will become apparent. Valuing and clarifying are the system processes used to answer these questions. Simply stated, as you ask if your moral-ethical behavior was right and responsible, you are both explicating and internalizing values.

Values Clarification

Values clarification processes deliberatively question the moral-ethical correctness or "rightness" of a decision. Values operating in moral-ethical comportment (and subsequently in ethical knowledge expressions) are often hidden. They can be thought of as the assumptions or background information that creates ethical-moral questions and moral-ethical moves. Our values direct us to see certain aspects of a moral problem and avoid others. Values vary among individuals and reflect the contexts of our experiences with family, friends, social institutions, gender boundaries, and age experiences. The questioning of values by using formal techniques of clarification assumes that values may not always be "good." It also assumes a disjunction between values we believe are operative in our actions and those that actually are.

There are various techniques for values clarification (Bandman, 1995; Davis, 1997; Simon, Howe, and Kirschenbaum, 1992; Steele, 1983; Wilderding, 1992), but fundamentally the processes involve the use of rational thought and emotional awareness to understand, examine, and actualize values. Approaches can use real or contrived dilemmas, group or individual work, self-analyses or interview, or any number of other methods that free individuals to examine and embrace their values. Clarification of values is often an emotionally charged activity involving deeply held personal beliefs. Individuals or groups undertaking values clarification processes need an environment that allows freedom of value choices and affirmation of the values clarified. Regardless of technique used, values clarification is an individualistic process that seeks to challenge and understand inculcated values. Values clarification is an important part of the valuing-clarifying process because it emphasizes affective thinking and behavior-motivated choice and allows one to question the responsibleness of moral-ethical decisions.

Various approaches for values clarification can be adapted to a specific situation. Some general guidelines, however, may be useful. First, it is important to select or create an ethical-moral dilemma that participants will emotionally relate to and not see as fictitious to their practice. Although commonly used approaches such as "which person to throw from the sinking boat" may suffice, more benefit is gained if the situations relate to actual or potential nursing practice. Second, focus on the explication of individual values that should emerge from the process, regardless of the process used for clarification. In values clarification there may be a tendency to avoid what is difficult. Lively discussions about what should be done do not substitute for a deliberative focus on one's personal values. A third guideline emphasizes writing about or listing personal values that emerge. Journaling around values not only helps explicate what the values are but also provides a forum for examining how and why values change. Because it is difficult to provide a public forum where learners can freely explicate and examine values, journaling becomes important—especially when the ethical-moral dilemmas that are the focus for deliberation arise from practice situations the participants are likely to encounter.

In values clarification some general questions that can be asked for a given situation include the following:

- What outcome would I like to see?
- What would I do?

- How do I feel about this? How strongly do I feel?
- What is guiding my potential actions? Feelings?
- What would need to change about the context for me to act or feel differently?
- Are there any alternatives in this situation, and how viable are they?
- How proud do I feel about my choices? Would I affirm them to others?
- Does there seem to be a hierarchy of choices?

Values Analysis

Another important process for questioning the moral-ethical correctness of a decision is values analysis. Unlike values clarification, which is an attempt to emotionally understand, clarify, and embrace individually held values, values analysis seeks to more objectively understand and analyze the values operating in a situation. In values analysis participants are required to recognize and stand apart from their own value structure as much as possible or see their value structure objectively and critically. In values analysis the participants strive to gain clarity on an issue, examine various points of view factually and logically, and examine different approaches to resolving the dilemma for empiric consistency and inconsistency. If factual evidence for one point of view is provided, it is questioned for accuracy. The ethical decision is arrived at logically, and then the decision is tested in some manner—for example, by looking at its consistency with a principle or code for ethical behavior. Values analysis is important because it points out the relativism and subjectivity of individual points of view. Like values clarification, the situations chosen for values analysis should arise from practice. Although explication of personal values is important in clarification, in analysis one looks at the values and justificatory processes that are operative in the situation. Rather than clarifying, What would I do? the questioning focuses on, What is going on? In values analysis the following questions may be used to guide discussion about a given situation:

- What are the ethical-moral issues?
- What ethical-moral decisions are being made?
- What ethical-moral bases are operating to guide those decisions?
- How strong are the arguments? The counterarguments?
- Is the evidence for the decisions truthful?
- Is more evidence needed to justify a decision? What sort?
- Are there any inconsistencies related to ethical decisions being made?
- What evidence do we need to know if the decisions are moral-ethical?
- What is the social and political context of the decision, and how is that affecting outcomes?

Both values clarification and values analysis are important processes for understanding the rightness and responsibleness of the ethical-moral decision making that will determine the nature of the knowledge form generated. The juxtaposition of personally cherished values (from values clarification) and objectively required values (from value analysis) deepens understanding of what is possible and what is necessary for nursing practice. When our value positions are challenged by an objective stance, they change. As the more objective value decisions are reached, we understand the limitations objectivism has in determining ethical-moral decision making.

The processes of values clarification and analysis include, whether recognized or not, reference to justice and care perspectives on ethical decision making, as well as reference to ethical theories, principles, and codes within the deontologic and teleologic perspectives. Within our model, then, valuing and clarifying processes—primarily values analysis and clarification—occur when questions of rightness and responsibleness are raised. Deliberate reflection of what is responsible and right may or may not occur; that is, the nurse involved in these processes may or may not deliberatively examine ethical knowledge forms as processes of clarification and analysis are accomplished.

ETHICAL KNOWLEDGE FORMS

The model we have created identifies principles and codes as ethical knowledge forms; however, other forms exist. Ethical knowledge may take the format of sets of rules; statements of duties, rights, or obligations; theories; or laws. The Nightingale Pledge (not created by Nightingale, we might add) and Hippocratic Oath are also forms of ethical knowledge. An individual nurse or group of nurses, setting forth an ethical position for disciplinary review out of values clarification and analyses processes, is likely to put it in the form of an article, a case analysis, or perhaps poetry. We have chosen principles and codes as generic forms of ethical knowledge because they are attainable and common forms of ethical knowledge in nursing. The American Nurses Association, for example, has created a code of ethics for nurses. Nurses are also taught to operate within are common forms of ethical knowledge such as principles of autonomy and beneficence. We also prefer to avoid associating ethical knowledge forms with "theory" to avoid confusion of the differences between ethical and empirical theories. Regardless of form of ethical knowledge, we suggest that eventually it can be reduced to principles and codes, which are shorthand ways of expressing ethical knowing.

DIALOGUE AND JUSTIFICATION

The disciplinary processes of dialogue and justification, like valuing and clarifying, require the collective and open examination of both behavior and knowledge. The model's central focus of moral-ethical comportment clearly suggests that the morality of practice and disciplinary ethical knowledge must be brought together. Notions of what is right and what is responsible not only question the moral-ethical dimensions of practice knowledge but also consider legal ramifications of practice as expressed in the language of rights and duty. In short, the ethics pattern embodies both epistemology and ontology through its focus on both ethics and morality.

It is within the model's processes of dialogue and justification that knowledge is more deliberatively examined with reference to established ethical theories, principles, codes, and the perspectives of justice and care. Through these processes ethical knowledge is examined and refined and becomes part of the disciplinary heritage that individual nurses subsequently carry into practice and revisit and challenge, with the use of the valuing and clarifying processes described previously.

Dialogue implies a community of askers who utilize established ethical perspectives, principles, and codes to accept, reject, or modify the knowledge form. Traditionally ethical knowledge forms are examined for an internal logic as a standard of validity. Although internal logic is important for coherence, it is an insufficient standard for establishing the value of ethical knowledge. Dialogue implies an ideal that multiple voices, over time, will be integrated into justificatory processes, whereas the choice of the word *justification* itself suggests no particular framework for establishing the value of an ethical knowledge form.

For dialogic justification of ethical knowledge forms in nursing, the justificatory templates that can be used include historical values associated with nursing, extant moral-ethical knowledge and currently held values, and values and moral knowing consistent with an envisioned future. For example, the value for caring might be cited as an important historical justificatory template for nursing—that is, caring as a historically embedded duty. Extant principles of nonmalevolence or autonomy, which baccalaureate students are universally exposed to, might be called up to justify ethical knowledge. Also, an envisioned future may form the critical template, as when we question whether caring is a ethic that will help us achieve professional autonomy and identity. It is assumed that the collective voice of nursing will be the best hope for the emergence of appropriate and productive justificatory templates as the basis for re-visioning the knowledge form.

We have chosen an eclectic approach to justificatory principles because we believe no one perspective is entirely useful for all situations. Rather, the more likely scenario is that multiple justificatory perspectives will be used. Care must be balanced with a concern for justice; rules must be used in the context of doing the least harm.

Suppose you are examining a case with a deontologic perspective that provides a rule for ethical action. Assume the rule asks you to be truthful and disclose fully. As the dialogue proceeds, the justificatory process takes a turn. Participants begin to realize that full disclosure may be counterproductive in some situations. Truth telling may conflict with another justificatory template, caring, or it may produce an awful lot of hurt. Which should prevail: the rule or caring? Should the rule be violated to produce a greater good? The answers are never clear-cut.

Although an eclectic approach to justification may seem to beg the question, the final template we would use to make decisions is the potential for the knowledge form to create a situation of praxis or reflective change. Ethical knowledge is often communicated in a vacuum, and we know little about how it is actually used or applied. Arguments for one type of approach versus another are academically interesting, but the truth is that there is much blurring about positions. For example, who can define what an ethics of care really is? It is through justificatory processes that a definition will be approached and ethical knowledge that is useful for praxis will emerge.

The justification and dialogue processes that are envisioned to evolve ethical knowledge are carried out over time, by multiple groups, with a variety of justificatory perspectives. These analyses and understandings will find their way into the disciplinary literature and other venues where dialogue can occur. It is ultimately through these processes, as is the case with other knowledge forms in nursing, that ethical knowledge forms will achieve a legitimacy in relation to practice. The ideal is to generate ethical knowledge from practice and to refine that knowledge with the intent that it will be returned to practice.

CONCLUSION

In this chapter we have considered the nature of ethics and morality, as well as processes for the development of disciplinary knowledge within the pattern of ethics. Ethical knowledge is developed when moral-ethical comportment as expressed in practice is questioned. The questions, Is this right? and Is this responsible? engage the processes of valuing and clarifying. From these processes ethical knowledge forms, including principles and codes, can be examined by members of the discipline by using the disciplinary processes of dialogue and justification. Ultimately, ethical knowledge is expressed as integrated moral and ethical comportment.

Reference List

Bandman EL: Nursing ethics through the life span, Norwalk, Conn, 1995, Appleton & Lange.

Carper BA: Fundamental patterns of knowing in nursing, Adv Nurs Sci 1:13, 1978.

Condon EH: Nursing and the caring metaphor: gender and political influences on an ethics of care, Nurs Outlook 40:14, 1992.

Cooper MC: Principle-oriented ethics and the ethic of care: a creative tension, Adv Nurs Sci 14:22, 1991.

Crowley MA: The relevance of Nodding's ethic of care to the moral education of nurses, J Nurs Educ 33:74, 1994.

Davis AJ: Ethical dilemmas and nursing practice, Norwalk, Conn, 1997, Appleton & Lange.

Fry ST: Toward a theory of nursing ethics, Adv Nurs Sci 11:9, 1989.

Gilligan C: In a different voice: psychological theory and women's development, Boston, 1982, Harvard University Press.

Hoagland SL: Some concerns about Nel Noddings' caring, Hypatia 5:109, 1990.

Houston B: Caring and exploitation, Hypatia 5:115, 1990.

Kohlberg L: Moral stages and moralization: the cognitive-developmental approach. In Lickona T, editor: Moral development and behavior: theory, research and social issues, New York, 1976, Holt, Rinehart & Winston.

Levine ME: The ethics of nursing rhetoric, Image J Nurs Sch 21:4.

Liaschenko J: Feminist ethics and cultural ethos: revisiting a nursing debate, Adv Nurs Sci 15:71, 1993.

Noddings N. Caring: *A Feminine Approach to Ethics and Moral Education*. Berkeley, 1984, Univ. of California Press.

Reverby SM: Ordered to care: the dilemma of American nursing, 1850-1945, Cambridge, 1987, Cambridge University Press.

Simon S, Howe L, Kirschenbaum H: Values clarification: a handbook of practical strategies for teachers and students, New York, 1992, Hart.

Steele SM: Values clarification in nursing, ed 2, Norwalk, Conn, 1983, Appleton-Century-Crofts.

Stewart IM: Some fundamental principles in the teaching of ethics, Am J Nurs 21:906, 1922.

Walker MU: Keeping moral space open, Hastings Center Report 23:33, 1993.

Wilderding JZ: Values clarification. In Gulechek G, McCloskey, editors: Nursing interventions: essential nursing treatment, Philadelphia, 1992, WB Saunders.

Chapter 8

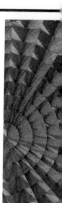

Personal Knowing

Self is a dynamic concept, ever deepening as we expand and broaden our relationships with others. The self is created in relation to others.

Beverly Hall and Janet Allan (1994, p. 112)

Personal knowing is the dynamic process of becoming a whole, aware self and of knowing the other as valued and whole. *Other* can be an individual, but small and large groups can also be known authentically and as a whole. Personal knowing is the basis for expression of authenticity, the genuine self, which in turn is essential in a healing relationship. Personal knowing expands that which is accessible to the self in the experience of the other; it enables experience of a deeper level of meaning shared in interaction.

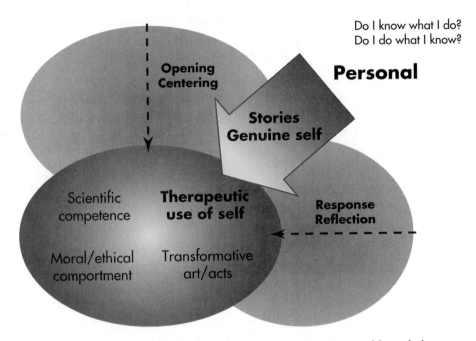

FIGURE 8-1 Processes for developing personal knowing and knowledge.

Figure 8-1 shows the personal knowing component of our model for knowledge development in nursing. In our model, personal knowing arises from the critical questions, Do I know what I do? and Do I do what I know? The processes of opening and centering create human capabilities of authenticity, the genuine self as well as autobiographic stories that provide a discursive form of expression of personal knowledge. These expressions of knowledge provide opportunities for response and reflection within the discipline. In practice, personal knowing is expressed as the therapeutic use of self.

In this chapter we explore conceptual meanings of personal knowing on which the processes of personal knowing are founded. We then provide descriptions of personal knowing processes that we have identified and used and that other nurse scholars have also identified and used. Within the descriptions of the processes we also explain the communicable forms of personal knowing that contribute to the development of personal knowledge within the discipline.

PERSONAL KNOWING IN NURSING

Personal knowing is fundamental to nursing by virtue of the nature of the interpersonal processes that are inherent to nursing practice. Personal knowing opens the way for being fully present with another, and interactions with others provide the experiential ground from which personal knowing emerges. As Hall and Allan (1994) state: "The self is created in relation to others" (p. 112). Personal knowing is the cornerstone upon which holistic practice in based, making possible wholeness of self and other in a context of relational experience (Hall and Allan, 1994).

The label *personal knowing* can be misleading in that it can imply a solitary and individual process, involving only the unique perceptions of the individual. Personal knowing involves deep inner reflection that is sometimes solitary, and it is an aspect of the whole of knowing that arises from within the individual. However, personal knowing also involves openness to experience in the world and with others and mutual, meaningful interactions with others. The contemporary popular notions of self-actualization and individuation reinforce images of the individual on a lone, often self-indulging journey of discovery (Hall, 1997). Moreover, contemporary cultures that value above all empiric knowing reinforce the mistaken notion that people are rational egos seeking individual autonomy, rights, and freedoms (Hart, 1997). Despite these dominant cultural contexts, personal knowing cannot be confined within the order of rational theory. The processes involved in personal knowing compel experience of the self as more than rational and as intimately connected to others.

Personal knowing is expressed as mind-body-spirit congruence, authenticity, and genuineness. Others experience and know the person as unique by virtue of those deeply personal qualities that are conveyed through being in the world and that express who the person is within the context of the culture. Personal knowing can also be conveyed through autobiographic stories, written or told, which provide a glimpse of who the person is in a form that is not confined to the time and space of the moment. Personal stories, like all other forms of discursive expressions of knowledge, are certainly limited in their capacity to convey the fullness of the person, but they provide a means of communication—and symbolically interacting with—a wide audience. This means of communication is vital within a discipline, where it is important to the discipline to create a shared understanding of what it means to know and develop the self. Discursive expression of personal knowing also opens opportunities for response from others and possibilities for deeper reflection.

CONCEPTUAL MEANINGS OF PERSONAL KNOWING

Carper's (1978) early description of personal knowing points directly to interpersonal interactions, relationships, and transactions as a central defining quality of nursing and to the fundamental necessity of personal knowing embedded in the concept of "therapeutic use of self."

> One does not know *about* the self; one strives simply to *know* the self. This knowing is a standing in relation to another human being and confronting that human being as a person. This "I-Thou" encounter is unmediated by conceptual categories or particulars abstracted from complex organic wholes. The relation is one of reciprocity, a state of being that cannot be described or even experienced—it can only be actualized. (Carper, 1978, p. 18)

For Carper, an authentic personal relation values others in their freedom to create themselves and make choices on their own behalf, which means setting aside generalizations and categories and assumptions taken from empiric forms of knowing, as well as manipulative, controlling, and impersonal forms of treatment. Instead, personal knowing embraces and values the wholeness and integrity in each encounter and seeks to know and affirm the uniqueness of each person and that person's unique experience.

Spirituality and Personal Knowing

Personal knowing is intimately related to spirit and to that which is sometimes referred to as spiritual (Bishop and Scudder, 1997; Hall, 1997; Hart, 1997; Huebner, 1985). The meanings of *spirit* and *spirituality* refer to the life journey of discovering personal meaning and purpose. *Spirit* is a term derived from the Latin word for "breath" and "breathing"; it conveys a sense of sustaining life, of an animating and vital principle inherent in Being (Huebner, 1985, p. 163). The "human spirit" is not something outside the person or a separate substance temporally residing within the body. It is the entirety of existence, and it is as spirits that people become most authentically themselves.

Spiritual is a term that is often linked with religion, a tradition that Hall (1997) identifies as deriving from the fact that Western culture limits expression of what is known either to science or to religion. Many people do connect their spirituality with religious beliefs. However, that which is spiritual does not of necessity link with any particular religious tradition. The spiritual is a complex of values, attitudes, and hopes that guide and direct a person's life. It is particularly linked to life experiences that bring one to the brink of uncertainty, the "existential boundary issues" of life and death, good and evil, hopes and dreams, despair and suffering. Personal knowing, taken as spirituality, means self-conscious awareness and nurturing of the interconnectedness of these life-challenging issues and also the inspiration to give shape to our lives as we confront them. Spirituality leads us to face the vulnerable realities of life that cannot be overcome and nurtures embodied spiritual agency for relating to these vulnerabilities (Hart, 1997).

Self-in-Relation

Hall (1997) presents a conception of human spirit and spirituality as reaching within to learn to accept, love, and value what we find there and learning to be ourselves authentically and with confidence. What we find within the spirit may not be what we want to find. It is the process of coming to know what is within, and coming to live with, accept, and love what is within is the process of personal knowing. This is not a process of self-centered exploration, nor is it linear. Rather, it is an unfolding process that is grounded in the context of everyday experience, in relationship with others.

Hall and Allan (1994) explain the vital link between personal knowing and relationships with others in their concept of self-in-relation. Their ideas are grounded in traditional Chinese medicine, which philosophically views mind, body, spirit, and environment as an integrated whole. The embodied self is seen as an open system that belongs to a social world. Self-in-relation is the core of caring and healing, of wholistic nursing practice. The caring relationships that nurses enter into can reflect four dynamics that nurture self-in-relation, as follows:

1. Caring by giving, which requires presence and involvement. In this process, mutual sharing develops the self and the other by giving to one another, affirming the value and purpose of each life.
2. Empowerment develops a sense of the self as responsible for health and ability to influence the health outcome. When the self is fully in relation with the other, both are empowered, and true unconditional love occurs. Both learn the joy of reciprocity, wherein what each brings to the interaction is deeply valued.
3. Knowing the value of a human life comes from a mutual quest to find meaning in life. In a healing relationship, questions of life and death, of living and dying, come to the surface, inviting an openness to explore what is possible in this particular time and space. Openness while fully engaging with another person in this quest develops the self in each.
4. Sense of community is the most important and most elusive concept in wholistic healing practice. A caring community that supports giving in interrelationships provides the context for developing self-in-relation.

Discovery of Self and Other

Moch (1990) defined *personal knowing* as the discovery of self-and-other arrived at through reflection, synthesis of perceptions, and connecting with what is known. She identified three overlapping components of personal knowing: experiential knowing, interpersonal knowing, and intuitive knowing. Experiential knowing is the understanding and knowledge that comes from participating in the events of daily living; it is deepened by attending to the experience, studying the process of the experience, and connecting the experience to previous understandings. Attending to the experience involves observing self and others and through feeling and sensing. For Moch, both cognitive and spiritual processes contribute to deriving meaning from experience. Interpersonal knowing is increased awareness through intense interaction or being-with another. It emerges from intense attending, opening self to other, and conveying feelings to another. Intuitive knowing is the immediate knowing of something without conscious use of reason.

Moch (1990) identified the following four attributes of personal knowing:

1. Personal knowing can be viewed only in the context of wholeness. There is no knowing apart from the knower.
2. Personal knowing includes a process of encountering. The ideal encounter is one of mutual respect, which affirms those involved in the encounter and their existence.
3. Personal knowing involves passion, commitment, and integrity. Passion is what affirms something as valuable, commitment motivates the search for personal meaning, and integrity brings thought and action together as an authentic whole.
4. Personal knowing involves a shift in connectedness or transcendence. This is the instantaneous "aha" experience in which one's perspective shifts, either consciously or unconsciously.

Unknowing

Munhall (1993) reflects Carper's point that knowing the other requires setting aside personal assumptions and generalizations. She stressed the nature of a genuinely authentic encounter by conceptualizing a pattern of "unknowing" to signify the existential openness to the other that must occur in such an encounter. Unknowing for Munhall creates a stance that is completely open to knowing the experiences and perceptions of others as they experience them, not filtered by the nurse's own structures of understanding. Unknowing means setting aside all that is assumed to be known about the other, as well as setting aside previously held organizing structures that make sense of the world—or "decentering" from the stance of the self to move into the life of the other. The nurse takes a deliberate stance of complete openness and receptivity to the unique subjectivity of the other and remains open to a deep knowledge of the other being, to different meanings and interpretations, and to varying perceptions of the world.

Despite certain distinctions in each of these conceptualizations of meaning, there are important threads that are common to the various conceptualizations. They include the primary importance of relationships and interactions in developing personal knowledge, an aspect of knowing that is beyond cognitive reasoning, the primacy of personal knowing in giving life its meaning and direction, and the imperative of wholeness and integrity that embraces the entirety of existence and experience. These common threads form the conceptual understandings on which our approaches to developing personal knowing are based.

PROCESSES FOR DEVELOPING PERSONAL KNOWLEDGE: OPENING AND CENTERING

In our model of knowledge development in nursing, the pattern of personal knowing stems from the questions, Do I know what I do? and Do I do what I know? Silva, Sorrell, and Sorrell (1995) pose the ontologic question, Who am I? and the epistemologic question, How do I come to know who I am? Each of these questions points to important aspects of the experience and the processes involved in developing personal knowing, with particular emphasis on the epistemologic aspects of how we come to know and express the whole, genuine self and the authentic being of the other.

Processes involved in developing personal knowing evolve in unique and individual patterns throughout a person's life, but there are dimensions of the experience of personal knowing that can be described. Personal knowledge in the discipline of nursing depends upon nurses' dedicated involvement in processes that contribute to their own personal knowing: sharing their insights with other nurses, engaging in mutual response and reflection to deepen their understanding of personal dimensions of knowing in practice, and developing abilities in the therapeutic use of self.

The ability to engage in a genuine authentic presence requires deliberate preparation and intent. Figure 8-2 depicts the interrelationships of preparation processes. Preparation involves private opening and centering practices over time that ground the individual in the center of the self (represented by the heart in the figure), so that the self is known, valued, assured, and loved by the self. Among the practices that can be used are journaling, meditation, various types of body-mind-spirit meditative practices such as yoga, and art forms. These practices bring mind-body-spirit into

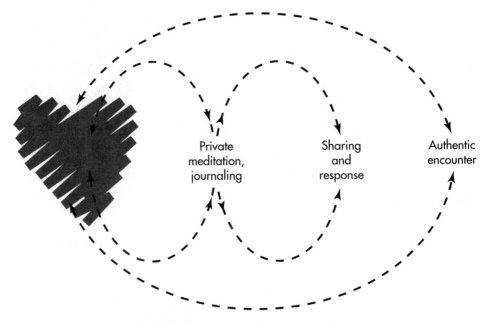

FIGURE 8-2 Preparation processes.

wholeness, create a time-space of inner calm and peace, and bring personal intentions and meanings to realization at a deep level that transcends consciousness.

From time to time, realizations that come from private centering practices enter into shared experiences with others and provide the opportunity to exchange responses, taking in new perceptions and reflections. As you return to your private time-space of centering, others' responses deepen and enrich your experience of self. In the figure the dotted loops, representing reflection, move through the private centering practices, back and forth between the heart center and the interactive responses of others, to depict the circular movement among the aspects of preparation. Preparation provides the core strength and character that enter into the authentic encounter, where the heart center of the person opens to be fully present with and for the other.

The preparation opening and centering practices of personal knowing are not "therapy." Therapy can assist a person in a quest for personal knowing, but it involves other purposes that focus on the compartmentalized mental or psychologic aspects of health. Preparation practices of personal knowing are integrated into daily life and focus on self-knowing as a whole, authentic being. Therapy involves an (often) unequal relationship in which one person provides therapeutic guidance and the other receives. In daily practices to nurture self-knowing, the individual reaches into an attentive mind-body-spirit center to come to know and love what resides within.

Opening and centering are interrelated processes that occur in many different ways and in as many different contexts. Opening and centering focus on lived experience and the meaning of that experience. They are processes that can emerge spontaneously and can be felt within experience, defying description or analysis. However, opening and centering occasions can be deliberately sought as individual, solitary processes that contribute to self-knowing (Beckerman, 1994). In the following section we discuss the practice of journaling and related meditative practices as examples of the elements of personal practice that nurture self-knowing and prepare the self for authentic encounters. Although we focus here on journaling and meditative practices, other forms of practice can be used in similar ways, depending on personal preferences.

Journaling and Meditation

Journaling, like other practices that nurture self-knowing, is a private encounter with the inner self. These practices require solitude away from other people and things. They require consistent, regular practice and time devoted to the practice. When you journal, what you write is never to be shared with others. Later, you can extract and revise segments from your journal with the intent of sharing with others, but the journal itself remains private to maintain your sense of safety for the expression of whatever feelings and perceptions emerge from deep within. In your journaling, you can let fears, anxieties, anger, and fantasies surface without even your own censoring. There are no critics peering into the inner self; even your own critical judgment is withheld as you seek to know and value your deepest self.*

Meditative practices can be used without journaling, but meditative practices are also a valuable part of journaling. As you settle into a time for journaling, begin by simply sitting still and quietly, turning your focus to your breath, and taking several deep breaths. Let the sense of your being settle into a centered space. You can move into the meditative practice of

---

*We stress this point for educators. We commend the use of journals for student learning and self-reflection, but when student journals are required to be shared with the teacher, the experience loses its fundamental value as a private, safe place where personal knowing can flourish. When journals are used as a teaching tool, we suggest helping students learn the value of this private form of personal growth. Sharing information from the journals can be a student's option, or students can be asked to excerpt material from their journals in a form of "public writing" that can be shared. See Nelson (1994) for further insights regarding the use of journals in teaching.

repeating a sound (mantra) or an affirmation that brings your focus closer to your center, to your deepest intentions, hopes, and desires. For example, you can repeat an affirmation such as "I trust my inner being" or "I am at peace with the path of my life."

When you feel ready, move to your journal to begin to bring your inner perceptions to the page. Journaling can include recounting facts and events, but move beyond the facts and events to explore how you feel and what is going on inside you. Likewise, as other people enter your reflections, move back to your own center and explore your sense of being in the situation and in relationship. Journaling is a process of working from both the conscious and the unconscious and of engaging in an inner experience with the self. The inner experience sensitizes your perceptions of events, people, and situations and brings you to a place of harmony and wholeness with who you are in relation to your world (Beckerman, 1994).

Abandon rules about written expression to fully express what you feel and your perceptions. You can doodle, draw, and let nonverbal images find expression on the page. Let the unexpected emerge without censorship or judgment. Imagine what you hope for and dream for, what your deepest desires are. If you feel drawn to analyze and judge what is coming forth, move back to nonverbal meditation, focus on your breath, and turn your attention once again to being open and feeling unconditional love and value for who you are. The time to analyze and rationally think through problems will come from your journaling process, and using this process to deepen your own inner sense of worth and self-love will give you greater clarity and strength to address problems. While you are meditating and journaling, always treat yourself as if you totally love yourself (Nelson, 1994).

You can enter into journaling with a specific intent, or you can enter the time-space with no particular intent other than to let your perceptions of your inner being come to the surface. If you are new to journaling or if you have had an experience or are involved in a situation that is saturating your consciousness, you can use a specific intent that focuses your journaling and meditation. The intent is not a problem-solving intent; rather, it is an intent to explore a particular aspect of your inner self. Box 8-1 gives an example of an intention that can be used to guide journaling.

Almost any image can be used as a focus for journaling as a means of using the process in ways that draw you into your inner self. Beckerman (1994) used works of art and focused her journaling on her perceptions of caring within the works of art. You can create an intention around your hopes and dreams, around memories, or around experiences. For example, you could write a prayer to express your deepest hopes and dreams. You could spend time journaling about different "selves" you have been throughout your life—your child self, your afraid self, your confident self. Typically, starting

Box 8-1

Intentional Journaling

Centering—Set your journal and your pen at your side. Find a comfortable position for your body. Let your breath flow in and out in a natural rhythm. As you breathe, let go of all tension in your muscles. Focus your attention on your inner experience—your feelings, hopes and desires, fears, or worries. Notice what aspect of your inner experience comes most fully to the surface.

Opening—For a few minutes, give this inner experience your full attention and let it come completely into your consciousness. Remain open to whatever comes to you, without judging or censoring your experience. Do not try to find solutions, or attempt to analyze the experience. Simply let the experience be, washing thoroughly through your mental awareness, your emotional feeling, and your physical sensations. You may need to laugh, cry, make sounds that match your experience, or move around to express what you are experiencing.

Journaling—Pick up your journal and your pen and put your experience in your journal. You may want to write words, or draw, or let the pen move in free form over the paper. Whatever your put in your journal, let it represent and describe your experience, just as it is.

Integrating—When you have finished journaling, set your journal and pen aside again and notice what your experience is like now. Notice your breath, any tensions in your muscles, your emotional and physical sensations. Notice what sounds or movements now seem to come to the surface.

Affirming—Find a word or phrase that now describes your inner experience and any shift that has happened in your experience. Place this word or phrase into an affirmation. For example, if you now feel released and free, you can use the affirmation "I am free to be." Write this affirmation in your journal, repeating it as many times as you are inspired to write it.

Returning—Take several deep breaths as you leave your journal and return to your usual activities. You can return again to your journal to explore other aspects of your inner experience, or to more fully explore this same experience. Notice how your experience shifts in both your usual activities, and in your journaling. From time to time, journal about the cycles and phases of your experiences.

with a focus simply opens doors and begins the journey to deep reflection, and the path of the reflection then moves in directions that transcend conscious intent.

PROCESSES FOR AFFIRMING PERSONAL KNOWING: RESPONSE AND REFLECTION

Response and reflection come from being in the world of experience with others. The self is perceived as unique by others; it brings to each situation and interaction a dynamic that is recognized and known. As people respond to one another, they give messages that affirm, disappoint, celebrate, or negate aspects of the expressed self. Responses are taken in, felt, and perceived. In processes of reflection, returning to meditative practices, the person reflects and takes in meanings that arise anew from the interactive experiences.

In addition to responses and interactions that happen in the course of daily experience, insights from meditation, journaling, and other self-knowing practices can be shared with trusted friends and colleagues who are willing to listen and respond to what is offered. Drew (1997), in exploring nurses' meaningful experiences and expanding self-awareness, found that sharing the story of experience with another enlarged, solidified, and deepened the meaning of the experience and gave the experience meanings that provided a guide for future interactions.

Autobiographic stories and short essays that are developed from your journal are a way of sharing insights that come to you from journaling while keeping your journal as a protected private document. What you share from your journal should be only what you are sure you want to share. You may have journaled feelings and emotions around a situation without writing the story of the situation. As you identify what you want to share, you might not include anything from your very personal journaling but use your journal to bring you back to the experience as you develop the story of the situation for sharing. Your journal will also draw you into deeper reflection as to the meaning of the situation, which you can weave into your story in language, metaphors, analogies or symbols. In some instances you may find excerpts that you do wish to extract and share or integrate into a written or verbal story (Nelson, 1994).

As formally developed autobiographic stories are developed and shared within the discipline, insights conveyed in the stories give others in the discipline an opportunity for reflection and response, which in turn enriches and deepens the personal knowing potential of others in the discipline. Although written stories are in one sense limited in their capacity to convey the essence of a person, they are rich in conveying inner processes and meanings that are not easily perceived in the interpersonal experience. Written stories provide opportunities for response and reflection that are different from those provided by the self alone.

FORMS OF EXPRESSION OF PERSONAL KNOWING

The genuine self, as Carper (1978) initially proposed, is the nondiscursive form of expression of personal knowing. The authenticity of the self is appreciated by the self and others, and it grows over time in interactions with others. Autobiographic stories provide a discursive form of expression of personal knowledge.

The aspect of practice that is known as the therapeutic use of self is the component of practice that arises from personal knowing. Therapeutic use of self can be discerned as a discrete aspect of a nurse's practice, but therapeutic use of self cannot be actualized without scientific competence, ethical-moral comportment, and transformative art-acts.

Formally developed autobiographic stories, written in the first-person voice of the nurse, provide a means of conveying personal knowing in a discursive form that can be widely communicated within the discipline. This type of well-developed story also reflects a dimension of aesthetics, but because it is written as a nurse's first-person account, it reveals deep personal insights and experiences that reveal personal knowing. Autobiographic stories also provide glimpses of ethical-moral comportment and scientific competence, but the main frame of the story remains within the realm of personal knowing.

The story in Box 8-2 was developed by Kathy Maeve from her personal reflections over weeks of caring for Dora. It speaks powerfully to her personal struggle to find meaning in the experience of being with Dora, of knowing Dora, and of caring for Dora. The story depicts caring for Dora, but the focus of the story is who Kathy is as a nurse caring for Dora—her own human experience as a nurse in relation to the caring experience. It is a story that speaks to other nurses and illustrates personal knowing.

Box 8-2

Regrets

To know Dora is to know regret. I regret the torture inflicted on her in the attempt to rid her body of this leukemia. I regret that we knew we couldn't. I regret the suffering she still has to go through as we finally allow the leukemia to take her life.

I regret that last night when I helped her to the bathroom, she very shyly covered herself, and wonder where such dignity comes from. I regret that because she cannot speak English, she has been treated like a little girl who cannot possibly know what is good for herself. I regret that the one time she acted for herself and boldly sneaked out of the hospital, everyone panicked and schemed about how to get her back. I regret that we did not honor her role as a mother and wife in a way that would have allowed her to realistically plan for these three small children she is leaving with a very young husband. I regret that he doesn't have a clue as to how to live without her.

Continued

Box 8-2

Regrets—cont'd

For myself, I deeply regret that I could not speak directly to Dora, but always had to rely on others. I deeply envied Carmen and Gunda's ability to easily talk with Dora, and Dora with them. But I was her advocate with the system—I ran interference for her. And I was very careful. I knew there was no room for mistakes or misjudgments. I was careful and deliberate. If I had not been so, Dora would have stayed in the hospital the entire last few weeks of her life. As it was, she was in and out on a regular basis but had some time alone with her husband and children. And Dora loved me for this. Still, Dora and Carmen and Gunda got to be women together, and I envied this most of all. Last night Dora told Carmen to tell me that she wishes she could have known me longer so she could have taught me to speak Spanish so the two of us could have "talked as friends."

The word "regret" hardly describes my sense of loss. So I have to make do with what I imagine about Dora. By my standards, she has had the worst of lives—20 years old, three children, an alcoholic husband who does not speak English and who has no real skills. Yet she had everything. For Dora was happy with who she was—so at home with her deep love for her children and for her husband too. And she had that beauty that young women have when they are full of love and passion and have their whole lives in front of them.

But we spoiled that beauty. We poked her body with needles at every opportunity. She lost her beautiful hair. She vomited so hard, and fried with fevers so high, we feared for her life continually. And then the leukemia finished off Dora's body. Her gums became infiltrated and grew over her teeth, giving her a somewhat gruesome smile. Her skin showed the signs of continual seeping of her precious blood into places where it could no longer sustain her life. And finally, she bled into her brain, shook before us, and never spoke or smiled again.

I look at her this night and see only her ashen body suffused with black and blue bruises and regret that such a beautiful young woman could ever look like this. I regret that all I can hear now is her bubbling breaths—her voice will never sound again. I regret that because of the loss of her silky black hair, her 2-year-old son calls her a "cuckooee." This is explained to me as a kind of monster, and I regret that any child of this Mexican Madonna could ever see her in this way.

So, finally, I pump morphine into her at increasingly high rates, for I cannot bear to feel that Dora is feeling anything. Her moans are stabbing at me. I want to run away instead of seeing her like this, yet I love her and I must be here—it must be me. So I go in and out of the room and cry with Carmen and Gunda over this sweet child that we cannot save but willingly nurse through this ugly death.

And it is ugly. I don't think I can bear it, yet I can't take my eyes away from Dora, or her year-old baby in the bed next to her, as he plays with his feet, blows bubbles, and smiles at everyone. He looks at Dora with certainty—he has seen Mommy sleep before.

From Maeve MK: The carrier bag theory of nursing practice, *Adv Nurs Sci* 16(4):19-20, 1994.

CONCLUSION

In this chapter we explored conceptual meanings of personal knowing upon which the processes of personal knowing are founded. We then provided descriptions of personal knowing processes that we have identified and used and that other nurse scholars have also identified and used. Within the descriptions of the processes, we also explained the communicable forms of personal knowing that contribute to the development of personal knowledge within the discipline.

Reference List

Beckerman A: A personal journal of caring through esthetic knowing, Adv Nurs Sci 17:71, 1994.

Bishop A, Scudder J: A phenomenological interpretation of holistic nursing, J Holistic Nurs 15:103, 1997.

Carper BA: Fundamental patterns of knowing in nursing, Adv Nurs Sci 1:13, 1978.

Drew N: Expanding self-awareness through exploration of meaningful experience, J Holistic Nurs 15:406, 1997.

Hall BA: Spirituality in terminal illness: an alternative view of theory, J Holistic Nurs 15:82, 1997.

Hall BA, Allan JD: Self in relation: a prolegomenon for holistic nursing, Nurs Outlook 42:110, 1994.

Hart H: Conceptual understanding and knowing other-wise: reflections on rationality and spirituality in philosophy. In Olthuis JH, editor: Knowing other-wise, New York, 1997, Fordham University Press.

Huebner DE: Spirituality and knowing. In Eisner E, editor: Learning and teaching the ways of knowing, Chicago, 1985, University of Chicago Press.

Maeve MK: The carrier bag theory of nursing practice, Adv Nurs Sci 16:9, 1994.

Moch SD: Personal knowing: evolving research and practice, *Sch Inq Nurs Pract 4:155, 1990*.

Munhall PL: "Unknowing": toward another pattern of knowing in nursing, Nurs Outlook 41:125, 1993.

Nelson GL: Writing and being: taking back our lives through the power of language, San Diego, 1994, LuraMedia.

Silva MC, Sorrell JM, Sorrell CD: From Carper's patterns of knowing to ways of being: an ontological philosophical shift in nursing, Adv Nurs Sci 18:1, 1995.

Chapter 9

Aesthetic Knowledge Development

> The first requisite [of nursing] is the practical belief that the greatest
> likeness among humans is their difference. The unspoken lesson
> of anatomy, the autopsy room, chemistry lab builds up the insidious
> biological impression of the body as a predictable entity—
> no wonder normal and alike become confused!
>
> *Katherine Brownell Oettinger (1939, pp. 1224-1225)*

Aesthetic knowing in nursing is that aspect of knowing that connects with deep meanings of a situation and calls forth inner creative resources that transform experience into what is not yet real, but possible. It is the dimension of knowing that connects with depths of human experience that are common but expressed and experienced uniquely in each instance. In practice the art of nursing is expressed in transformative art-acts. Formal expression of aesthetic knowledge takes the forms of aesthetic criticism and works of art.

Figure 9-1 shows the aesthetic knowing component of our model for knowledge development in nursing. In our model the aesthetic pattern of knowing in nursing poses questions such as, What does this mean? and How is it significant? Silva, Sorrell, and Sorrell (1995) pose the ontologic question, What does my perceptual sensibility to art reveal to me? and the epistemologic question, How do I come to know the artistry? From these questions the processes of envisioning and rehearsing nurture artistic

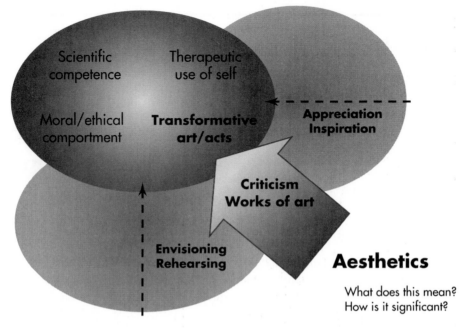

FIGURE 9-1 The aesthetic component of knowledge development in nursing.

expression of aesthetic knowing. The discursive form of aesthetic knowing is criticism; works of art such as poetry, stories, and photographs are nondiscursive forms of expression of aesthetic knowing that provide for the discipline a source of appreciation and inspiration. In practice, aesthetic knowing is expressed in transformative art-acts, in which the nurse moves experience from what is to a new realm that would not otherwise be possible.

In this chapter, we begin with a discussion of the meaning of art and aesthetics as background for the conceptualization of art and aesthetics in nursing. Next we present a conceptual definition of the art of nursing and discuss our definition in light of other conceptualizations of the art of nursing that have appeared in nursing literature. Finally we focus on the epistemologic dimensions of ways to develop aesthetic knowing and knowledge. These methods also incorporate important dimensions that address the ontologic processes of experiential perceptual sensibility.

ART AND AESTHETICS

Aesthetics is a noun that derives from the Latin and Greek words referring to perception. It has evolved to refer specifically to the perceptual ability to appreciate artistically valid form. The adjective *aesthetic* identifies an object or experience as artistically valid. That which is artistically valid is coherent in form and substance, conveys meaning of a whole beyond the formative and substantive elements, and evokes a response.

The standards by which something is taken to be artistically valid vary widely in different disciplines and in different contexts. Individuals, given their unique perceptions and tastes, respond differently to an aesthetic object or experience. However, within a given community or discipline, the cultural-disciplinary heritage and explicit or implicit collectively derived criteria of worth place the individual within a frame of reference that mediates the perception of artistic validity. Regardless of individual or culturally derived responses, that which is taken to be artistically valid can be recognized as placing various elements into a pattern to form a whole that symbolizes meaning beyond the elements themselves and that evokes a feeling response.

Ordinarily aesthetics is associated with art. However, things that may not be ordinarily labeled as art have aesthetic characteristics (Sandelowski, 1995). A scientific theory, for example, is a creation that is formed from the elements of conceptual ideas into a pattern that conveys a meaning that the concepts taken alone could not convey. The appeal (a subtle feeling response) of a theory often derives from the aesthetic shape of the theory, its coherence. Without this quality the theory lacks a certain attractiveness or appeal to the community of scientists.

Art is the process of creating an aesthetic object or experience; it is also the term used to refer to the product that is created. Art as a process involves acquired skill in technical and mechanical aspects of working with the elements from which the product is formed, as well as inner capacities to imagine the whole before it becomes an expression and to intuitively bring into being the elements as an integral whole. This process can be readily illustrated in the fine arts, where, for example, the musician acquires technical and mechanical skills with an instrument and learns to bring the elements of sound into expression as a whole musical rendition that generates particular responses for the listener. Art as a product is a form that gives rise to feeling and transforms experience. Art draws the person (whether observer or participant) into a realm that would not otherwise be accessible to experience. Art expands perceptual capacities and possibilities.

Art is not limited to the fine arts. Art is present in all human activity that involves forming elements into a whole. The extent to which the process is satisfying—and the product assumes coherence as a whole that elicits a feeling response—defines the extent to which the experience can be called "art" (Eisner, 1985). Value judgments of the worth of any artistic expression do not define something as "art"; that is, art is not limited to that which is called "good art" by some external standard. In many contemporary cultures, what can be called art has come to mean that which will sell or bring a profit. To the contrary, art is found in everyday experience and in multitudes of forms of expression.

Likewise, aesthetic qualities (elements placed into a pattern to form a whole, symbolizing meaning beyond the elements themselves) can be reflected in all aspects of nursing practice—from notes written in a chart to theoretic formulations, from a single brief interaction with an individual to sustained interactions with groups and communities, and from an unexpected encounter to a thoughtfully planned design for a system of care. In all of these ranges of nursing experience, nurses draw on and use science, ethics, and personal knowing, as well as aesthetic knowing; it is the dimension of aesthetic knowing that endows the experience with its aesthetic qualities.

In philosophy aesthetics addresses the nature and expression of beauty. Beauty is not taken to mean strictly that which, as a matter of taste, is perceived to be beautiful. Rather, it is that which takes a form that satisfies or appeals. The substance of that which is addressed as "beauty" in philosophy may, in fact, represent something like sorrow, pain, or despair, but the form of expression conveys a sense of wholeness, a goodness of fit, congruity, integrity, rhythm, harmony, or flow. Regardless of substance, the form reflects characteristics of congruence or fit to form a whole. As Carper (1978) stated in her early explanation of the aesthetic pattern of knowing in nursing, "The design, if it is to be esthetic, must be controlled by the perception of the balance, rhythm, proportion and unity of what is done in relation to the dynamic integration and articulation of the whole" (p. 18).

Aesthetic knowing has two components: knowledge of the experience toward which the art form is directed and knowledge of the art form itself. For example, the poet requires knowledge of a life experience that is reflected in the poem, as well as knowledge of the techniques and methods used to create something that can be called poetry. The visual artist requires knowledge of the experience or situation that will be visually presented on a canvas, as well as knowledge of the technical aspects of painting, to achieve the desired visual symbols and representations.

In nursing knowledge of experience encompasses knowledge of the *experience* of nursing and the *experiences* of health and illness. It is the lived experience of nursing, and of health and illness, toward which our aesthetics is directed, and it is the experience itself that our art is intended to transform. Background knowledge of experience is acquired through education, through hearing or reading stories about experience, and from experience itself. Nurses learn, for example, about the experience of dying by studying theories of death and dying, by reading or hearing stories about dying, and by caring for people who are dying and their loved ones. Immediate knowledge of experience comes from experiencing another's feelings (Carper, 1978). It involves empathy but includes intuitive knowing and all other possible modes of perceiving another's reality, some of which may not yet be named.

Knowledge of nursing's art form itself is the focus of this chapter. We will explore a definition of the art of nursing, the elements that form the whole of the art as a product, the technical skills involved in creating the art-act, and the processes by which those elements can be shaped to form a satisfying, artistically valid whole. The conceptualization of the art of nursing and of the processes that bring the art of nursing into being forms the foundation for developing knowledge of the art form. From this foundation, we describe the processes involved in developing aesthetic knowledge in nursing.

CONCEPTUAL DEFINITIONS OF THE ART OF NURSING

As Johnson (1994, 1996) demonstrates, the idea of the art of nursing has had several different meanings reflected in nursing literature since the time of Nightingale. Although no single clear definition of the art of nursing prevails, nurse scholars have consistently recognized a phenomenon they name "the art of nursing" and believe that this aspect of nursing is vital to who nurses are and what they do. A large part of the difficulty in specifying "the art of nursing" is related to the fact that it resides in an ontologic plane; it is expressed in the being-knowing of the nurse. In this realm it does not seem reasonable or possible to fully separate that which can be viewed as aesthetic from that which can be viewed as other patterns of knowing. We can recognize aspects of being that clearly reflect aesthetic form and structure, but these are closely intertwined with scientific competence, therapeutic use of self, and ethical-moral comportment.

Another ontologic dimension that contributes to the difficulty in specifying "the art of nursing" is the embodied nature of art. Art is directed toward the transformation of experience. Human experience is a body-mind phenomenon in which the dichotomies that prevail in the conventional construction of knowledge cannot be sustained. The project of defining a concept and developing knowledge is typically placed within the conventional tradition, where the rational mind prevails.

Recognizing the challenges derived from the ontologic dimensions of the aesthetic, of the whole, for this discussion we shift focus to the epistemologic question posed by Silva, Sorrell, and Sorrell (1995): How do I come to know the artistry? To address this question, it is necessary to conceptually define the phenomenon of the art of nursing as precisely as possible, integrating understanding of the ontologic dimensions of art. The definition of the art of nursing that we offer here was derived from discussions with practicing nurses who, without exception, recognized meaning in the phrase "the art of nursing" and provided rich discussion of their practices associated with this idea (Chinn, 1994; Chinn, Maeve, and Bostick, 1997). The inquiry drew on observations of nurses as they practiced nursing, photographs of the nurses as they practiced, journaling to explore deeper symbolic meanings of the practices observed, discussions and storytelling among nurses concerning their experiences of the art of nursing, discussions of possible story lines elicited by viewing the photographs, and rehearsals of aesthetic elements (movement and narrative) of nursing practice as these components took shape. The definition that emerged from this inquiry is as follows:

> The nurse's synchronous arrangement of narrative and movement into a form that transforms experiences into a realm that would not otherwise be possible. The arrangement is spontaneous, in-the-moment, and intuitive. The ability to make the moves that are transformative is grounded in a deep understanding of nursing, including relevant theory, facts, technical skill, personal knowing, and ethical understanding; and this ability requires rehearsal in deliberative application of these understandings. (Chinn, Maeve, and Bostick, 1997, p. 90).

This definition identifies synchronous narrative and movement as the elements that nurses use in forming the aesthetic experience—which is what in this book we call the transformative art-act. Synchrony is taken to mean the sense of coordination and rhythm of the engaged experience. It is also taken to mean the symbolic synchrony of intention and action coming together as an integral whole.

Synchronous narrative and movement as the elements that form the aesthetic in nursing is a critical feature of the Chinn, Maeve, and Bostick (1997) definition (which we are also using for the purposes of this chapter) that has not appeared elsewhere in the nursing literature. As we show later in this chapter, conceptualizing the elements from which nursing art is formed provides substance to understanding and developing knowledge of the art form itself. Other aspects of this definition are connected to the meanings of the art of nursing that Johnson (1994) identified in the nursing literature, but our definition also conveys important distinctions. The following sections present the distinct conceptualizations of the art of nursing that Johnson identified in nursing literature and discussion of the Chinn, Maeve, and Bostick (1997) definition in light of these prior conceptualizations.

The first distinct meaning for nursing art that Johnson identified in the literature is *nursing art* as the ability to grasp meaning in patient encounters. In our definition of the art of nursing, the ability to grasp meaning in a complex nursing situation toward which our art form is directed is implied, in that a grasp of meaning in a situation is required if the nurse is to transform an experience from what is to what might be possible. In Johnson's (1994, 1996) interpretation of prior conceptualizations of the ability to grasp meaning, it is the meaning of the situation that is perceived intuitively and in the moment; that is, the intuitive aspect is engaged to perceive the health-illness experience of those for whom we care (the experience toward which our art is directed). In our definition explicit reference to the intuitive, in-the-moment dimension refers to the intuitive element of the art form itself, not to the experience toward which nursing art is directed. This does not mean that immediate grasp of the situation itself does not also occur. Rather, the focus for defining the art form of nursing resides in the intuitive use of creative resources to form experience. The nurse is open to making moves within an experience that might not have been anticipated and planned but rather moves that come from a perceptual grasp of the formative possibilities that reside within the experience and that come from a creative wellspring within the nurse's art-as-process. The intuitive aspect of creating form is what we typically refer to as creativity. It is a knowing-in-the-moment-of-creating that enables the artist to express unique possibilities that fit, that fall into the whole in right relationship. It then follows that intuitive perception of right relationship within the form depends, in a nursing encounter, on a deep grasp of meaning embedded in the situation.

Prior conceptualizations that concern the ability to grasp meaning either explicitly or implicitly refer to meaning in patient encounters. Our definition is clearly applicable to patient encounters but can also be found in nursing actions that do not involve a direct patient encounter. The ability to design a system of care (for example, the system of care designed by Lydia Hall; see Chapter 2) is grounded in a grasp of meaning in the experience of people for whom the system is designed. Here, the spontaneous and intuitive aspect of the process of creating the design occurs in the formation process, where the nurse designer is immersed in the experience of creating the design and is open to the flow of possibilities that emerge as the design takes shape.

The second conceptual meaning that Johnson (1994) identified in the nursing literature is the ability to establish a meaningful connection with the patient. This aspect of the art of nursing is implied in our definition rather than explicit, in that "transformative moves" require a connection of a certain type. This is closely related to the ability to grasp meaning in a situation; without a grasp of meaning, a meaningful connection is not possible. Transformative moves require presence with the other, literally or symbolically. In the context of relationship, synchronicity or rhythmicity can be perceived. The "synchronous arrangement of narrative and movement" elicits a synchronous interaction, with a timing and flow among all elements, including those present in the situation. The observable synchronicity symbolizes the deeper level of connection between the nurse and the patient and is symbolic of the meaning in the connection.

The third conceptual meaning for the art of nursing that Johnson (1994) identified is the ability to skillfully perform nursing activities, which is one of the earliest conceptualizations of nursing art and a meaning that was often expressed by nurses who participated in Chinn's (1994; Chinn, Maeve, and Bostick, 1997) aesthetic inquiry. Nurses first pointed to tasks and procedures that are required in the "doing" of nursing, noting that it is *how* they do what they do that characterizes their art. The skills themselves do not constitute the art of nursing. Rather, the ability to "skillfully perform" is a characteristic of aesthetic form expressed in the nature of the nurse's movement and narrative, which may or may not involve tasks and procedures. Skillful performance derives from a background of rehearsal that makes possible what Benner and Wrubel (1989) identify as "ready-to-hand" knowing. In our definition skillful performance is explicit with respect to technical skill. However, the definition implies an integration of technical skill with relevant theory, facts, personal knowing, and ethical understanding, and the rehearsal that is required to develop the art of nursing is an integrated form of rehearsal in which all dimensions of being and acting are brought together to form a whole.

The fourth conceptual meaning that Johnson (1994, 1996) identified is the ability to rationally determine an appropriate course of nursing action. Recent work concerning clinical judgment and reasoning (Benner, Tanner, and Chesla, 1996; Mattingly and Fleming, 1994) recognizes the intuitive and aesthetic components that are necessary for sound practice. However, in our conception rational judgment is not a defining element of the art of nursing. In our definition rational ability, like technical skill, is background necessary to aesthetic capability. It constitutes an important component of knowledge of that toward which nursing art is directed, but it does not point to knowledge of the art form itself. The artist must draw on rational understanding in the process of artistic creation, but rational understanding is not the key element of aesthetic sensibility. A composer, for example, applies accepted theories of rhythm in constructing a musical score but in the process has spontaneous, intuitive inspiration to integrate rhythmic variations that may defy common conventions. In so doing the composer places a unique signature on the work that gives it artistic value and character. Likewise, the nurse applies theoretic understanding of a particular type of illness experience in developing a rational plan of care to point toward appropriate nursing action but remains open to spontaneous and intuitive inspiration to integrate variations as the caring process unfolds. It is the variations integrated with rational understanding that signify artistic form, and the particular ways in which the nurse shifts or moves through the experience convey an artistic signature, a particular and unique quality to the experience.

Finally Johnson identified the ability to morally conduct one's nursing practice as a distinct conceptual meaning of the art of nursing that has appeared in the nursing literature. Like technical skill and rationality, our definition of the art of nursing points to ethical understanding as background essential to aesthetic practice. There is a value component in the idea of "transformative moves" that implies a significant ethical dimension inherent in the art of nursing, in that transforming creates a change in what would otherwise be. Nurses who participated in the aesthetic inquiry from which our definition was derived told many stories of their practice that involved ethical dilemmas and that elicited actions that they associated with the art of nursing. Although it can be said that an experience could not be recognized as artistically valid if it violates ethical sensibilities, aesthetic knowledge in itself does not convey ethical understanding (Vezeau, 1994). Rather, aesthetic representation can reveal the significance of ethical and moral dilemmas and contribute to developing ethical sensibilities (Maeve, 1994). The ethical component that can be identified within the art of nursing comes from the integration of ethical comportment and transformative art-acts.

PROCESSES FOR DEVELOPING AESTHETIC KNOWLEDGE

The processes for developing aesthetic knowledge are envisioning possibilities, rehearsing, and forming the elements of the art into perceivable reality by creating representations of the possibilities. From these creative processes, aesthetic criticism can be constructed that reveals a discursive form of knowledge of the artistry of nursing. Works of art also emerge as representations of what is known, providing a nondiscursive means of representing aesthetic knowledge to the broader audience of the discipline. Art forms that have been created in nursing to represent the meaning and significance of nursing and health experiences include poetry, photography and other visual art forms, story, drama, and dance (Chinn and Watson, 1994).

As nurses share and communicate insights derived from the processes of envisioning, rehearsing, and representing the artistry of nursing, the responses of others in the discipline place the work and the meanings represented within the context of the discipline. The connoisseur processes of appreciation and inspiration reflect back on the experience that is represented, the representations, and the symbolized meanings that are conveyed through the representations. Connoisseur processes deepen shared knowledge of the art of nursing.

Transformative art-acts are the nondiscursive, ontologic expression of the art of nursing in nursing contexts. These art-acts are characterized by synchronous forms of movement and narrative that transforms the health-illness experience from what is into a realm that would not otherwise be possible. These art-acts usher the experience of those involved from one moment to the next, expanding the realm of possibilities into the future (Benner and Wrubel, 1989). In these instances everything comes together in synchrony, like a dance. It "works" for everyone involved in the situation. This experience has an element of mystery; it is perceived in the moment but not consciously or analytically understood. It involves feeling moved to a realm of possibility that had not been planned or anticipated but that is sensed as right for the moment.

Envisioning and Rehearsing

Envisioning and rehearsing are two interrelated processes from which creative possibilities emerge and within which aesthetic knowing is grounded. They are processes that can be perceived when nurses describe their art, for nurses who have acquired artistic capacity have intuitively engaged in these processes in the course of their nursing practices. They have not been deliberately taught, nor have they conceptualized what they do in this way. In fact, many of the practices that we came to view as envisioning and rehearsing (Chinn, Maeve, and Bostick, 1997) involve activities that the nurses hid from view, engaged in their off hours, and previously assumed to be insignificant and trivial yet sometimes necessary to cope with difficult situations. For example, as nurses described situations that represented their art, they consistently also related how they told one another stories about the situation in phone conversations after work, over a meal, or in a secluded area during a down time. Their storytelling episodes always included an account of the response of the listener and the way their interactive talk formed and re-formed how they came to see similar situations and how they came to trust their own intuitive senses. When we associated these and similar activities as a necessary and important aspect of developing aesthetic knowing of their art form, the nurses immediately grasped the connection.

A useful frame for understanding the processes of envisioning and rehearsing is that of improvisation. In an improvisational art, which characterizes the art of nursing, the display (or performance) is possible because of carefully developed skills in the various moves and sequences that can be called forth in any unique situation. This requires intense rehearsal and development of finely tuned skills that are fully embodied. The artist develops skills covering a wide range of possible effects or feelings that the improvisation might call for and rehearses imagined passages before a coach or critic to receive direction concerning the symbolic meanings conveyed in each passage. For example, in improvisational drama the actor develops sequences of movements, postural and facial expressions, voice intonations that convey wide ranges of emotion, and narrative lines that give verbal expression to possible experience. The director (critic, coach, teacher) gives the artist feedback and guidance that leads the actor into new territory at times or guides the actor through repeated trials of an emerging sequence to perfect the sequence and bring the moves to a refined, embodied level. When, in the improvised interaction on stage, a particular attitude emerges, the actor has the skills so finely tuned that in the improvised moment, the actor's focus remains in the moment of the interaction and on the process that is emerging in the improvised situation. The actor does not convey authenticity if the moves are not fully embodied; the actor cannot pretend (a notion often associated with "acting"). Rather, authenticity can come only from moves that have become so fully embodied that the actor thoroughly feels and experiences the situation.

In the following sections we describe the processes for envisioning and rehearsing narrative and movement as elements of nursing practice. The processes we describe are not linear or sequential. Any one process can be the particular focus for a time, but they most often come together and interweave. They are presented separately here to describe in some detail what they are and how they function to contribute to aesthetic knowing. The processes include (1) creating and re-creating story lines, (2) creating and developing embodied synchronous movement abilities, and (3) rehearsing a situation and engaging a critic.

Creating and Re-Creating Story Lines. When nurses tell stories to one another, they move into a realm that is created from the imagination and is not bound by the constraints of the workaday world. Even when the story begins with the intention of conveying an accurate account of a real experience, in the telling of the story the narrator creates emotion, stresses points of emphasis, exaggerates or downplays selected elements of the story, and selects certain features to include or exclude. Often the desires of the storyteller peek through in ways that surprise even the storyteller. Unexpectedly the storyteller gives, for example, an account of what she or he wishes had been done in the situation as if it actually happened, rather than accounting for what did happen. If the story were viewed through the lens of empirics, the story would have little or no worth. Viewed through the lens of aesthetics, the story has exquisite value as a frame from which to explore possible avenues of understanding and meaning, to shift experiential ground and expand perceptual capabilities called forth by the new ground, and to create visions and possibilities for the future (Maeve, 1994).

A story that is grounded in aesthetic knowing is told in the voice of the person who receives nursing care. The story illuminates the experience toward which nursing's art form is directed while it also portrays elements of the character of the art form that is conveyed by the nurse in the story. The story can come from actual experience, but aesthetic storytelling does not require adhering to the factual "truth" of a situation, as an empiric case study or anecdotal account requires. The storyteller purposely exaggerates, fictionalizes, emphasizes, and reshapes the actual experience to enhance listeners' perception of certain meanings that are intended to be conveyed in the story. The story comes from the imagination more than from the actual experience, although the imagination is often inspired by actual experience. The well-developed story will reveal a deeper truth of insight, understanding, and wisdom, the deepest meanings and possibilities in human experience, which are often not manifested in empiric reality or perceived cognitively.

In the process of creating of a story line, the essential characters are placed in a situation that presents a tension that moves toward an uncertain ending. The story line might be based on an actual situation, the ending of which is known, but for the purposes of aesthetic development the ending is left open and variable. The tensions that move toward the ending are central to the process of creating different story lines. Characters other than the essential characters can shift and move in and out of the story; each character can take on different roles as the story lines shift.

Creating and re-creating story lines serves several purposes related to aesthetic knowing. Most important from the perspective of aesthetics, each story line brings forth new perceptions of meaning that could be possible in the situation. The varying story lines bring to awareness how various meanings are symbolized in human experience and open new possibilities for creative engagement with each emerging meaning. Stories elicit profound reflection on meaning, both personal meaning and the meanings that others represent in the story. In this way story brings to awareness knowledge of that toward which our art is directed—the experiences of those for whom we care and the meanings that can be embedded in those experiences.

Creating and re-creating story lines also provide narrative experience and rehearsal, which in turn develop knowledge of and skill with the art of nursing itself. Creating story lines provides felt experience of placing intention into action as an integral whole. It also provides rehearsal of integrating present possibilities within the frame of past and future. The exact words that emerge in the process of creating and re-creating story lines are not those used in the actual practice situation, but the facility to form narrative lines develops the facility to use narrative effectively in practice. The narrative that is used to tell a story places the plot within a context; conveys the "feel," the attitude, and the mood of the story; and integrates the various elements of the story line to form a whole vicarious experience placed in narrative time and space. Narrative that is used in practice serves the same functions, in that it places the isolated real experiences of the person into a larger plot, contributes to creating an atmosphere within which the experience unfolds, and integrates the various elements of experience into the whole of the past, present, and imagined future. In the rehearsal of creating and re-creating story lines, you work with complete or nearly complete narratives. In practice the complete story line may never unfold, but the narrative moves of the nurse serve to shift experience into and through an emerging life plot.

In creating a story line you can develop your ideas in writing (Sorrell, 1994) or in conversation. The creation of a story line can begin with an anecdotal account of a real experience. The experience can be your own, or it can be an experience that you observed or have heard about. The first account of the experience is likely to seem relatively simple and inadequate to represent the significance of the experience itself, and it may sound "clinical" because of the culturally acquired propensity to recount clinical case studies. To create a story line, first explore what about this experience compels your attention, identify the key characters involved in the experience, and imagine each character's perspective, motives, and intentions. Explore the context within which the experience was set and key elements of the situation that seem important to the unfolding of the story. Imagine various endings toward which your experience could have moved or might move. Ultimately you will select a preferred ending, but various endings provide possibilities for building tensions within the middle of the story around what is possible and toward uncertain endings.

Next sketch out the essential characters that you wish to place within your story line. You can shift the characters as your story line unfolds and changes, but the characters will remain central to the story line. As you sketch the characters, the elements of the story line will begin to emerge because characters change over story-line time. Imagine several different possibilities for the movement of the story line, and let one of the possibilities emerge into the story. This will be your first narrative, material with which you can work in re-creating the story line with other possible endings.

Five principles associated with creating and re-creating story lines (Mattingly, 1994) are as follows:

1. The interactions between the characters of the story and their motives provide key structuring devices. Unlike clinical accounts of illness, a story line shifts attention away from the contingencies of the illness, disability, or health challenge to the way the characters in the story structure their experiences. Actions, interactions, and motives move the story line along toward the end of the story without revealing the end.

2. The story line is organized within a time-space of desire, where what is happening as the story unfolds is a time-space that cannot remain static because it is a place where the characters and others drawn into the story do not want to be. The story line compels movement toward an ending and elicits a desire for an ending even in the listener or reader of the story. The valence of desire elicits an unexpected account of what the nurse wishes she or he had done, rather than what actually was done, in telling a story.

3. Change is central to a story line. People and things change over time. Time moves toward an end, but within the line of the story, time can play tricks of reversal and circularity, boomerang around, and cross time lines situated before the story begins. The ending of the story represents a transformation from the state of affairs at the beginning of the story, and the agency that is the most important in creating the transformation is human motive and action.

4. Conflict, struggle, and tension are ever present. The beginning of a story line sets up the focus of the tension, and as the story line proceeds, the obstacles to be overcome in dealing with the tension unfold. The story line simultaneously builds the desire to resolve the tension. As the story line moves forward, the voices of the key players express different perspectives on the tension and the desired ending and leave the ending uncertain.

5. Endings remain uncertain throughout the story line, sometimes even through the ending of the story. Several different anticipated endings never happen. As the story line unfolds, what is positioned between the past (the beginning) and the future (the end) is a landscape of what is possible. The ending of the story need not be logically necessary, but rather it illustrates what is possible. The ending of the story line must be plausible, but it is only one of several plausible endings.

These same features characterize the story that unfolds in real life for a person experiencing illness, disability, or other health challenges (Mattingly, 1994). The difference is that the story unfolds in small increments placed in experienced time. The interactions, motives, and intentions of the people involved in the situation are the key structuring device that develops the plot of the story and moves the real-life story forward. What is happening is usually not a place the key players desire, or they know they cannot stay in this place (like the moments after the joyful birth of a child). The desire to move forward and to move into a different place is strong. Change is central; every day—sometimes every moment—brings with it a new challenge. Conflict, struggle, and challenge are ever present, and there are obstacles to be overcome. The ending of the story remains uncertain, with the unfolding life story positioned between the past and the future, where the landscape is what is possible.

Creating and re-creating story lines provide aesthetic narrative skills that the nurse uses as a participant in the emerging real-life stories of those cared for. The experienced unfolding story is shaped and transformed by the emerging possibilities of the present time situated between past and future. Mattingly (1994) describes this process as "therapeutic emplotment." The story that unfolds is not constructed in the same way a story line is constructed and is usually not told as an explicit story. Instead, the plot of the story is lived. The aesthetic challenge is to gradually structure isolated episodes into a plot that moves toward a possible end and bring to the experience actions and narrative lines that emplot the experience and that move the experience toward a possible ending. The synchrony among all the participants of the real-life story signifies their mutual participation in the creation of the plot, the selection of a possible ending, and the creation of the shifts of action that bring about changes and transformations as the lived story unfolds. The plot unfolds in moment-by-moment interaction; it cannot happen as a plan or a design. The possible desired end toward which the participants wish to move provides a force toward which movement is directed. The nurses' ability to participate in this essentially aesthetic process is nurtured by skills they develop through rehearsal in creating and re-creating story lines.

Creating Embodied Synchronous Movement. Movement is inherent to the practice of nursing, and yet very little attention is given to systematic development of movement skills, other than body mechanics. Movement is taken for granted; people enter nursing with a lifetime of experience in moving through space and with a cultural understanding of the symbolic significance of various moves, gestures, and postures. Within the frame of the art of nursing, movement takes on a very different level of significance. Movement is a body-mind-heart integrity, where what is expressed in a body move represents a complex flow of intention, concerns, hopes, desires, and fears.

As an element of the art of nursing, movement becomes the medium for expression of meaning that parallels visual representation in the arts. Like the picture that conveys a thousand words, the movements of the nurse express a multitude of meanings, at many levels of depth. The communicative power of movement includes what is popularly known as body language, sending messages grounded in the culture that require no language and, in fact, at times defy language. In addition, movement communicates who the nurse is, the nature of the nurse's intentions, how the nurse regards the self, the genuineness of the nurse, the nurse's capacity for being in relationship, and the nurse's level of technical and scientific competence.

Movement, including posturing, engages synchronous interaction. How the nurse moves in and around a situation sets a rhythm, a style, a dynamic, a pace, and an attitude that invites engagement and entrainment. It is a fundamental symbolic marker of the synchronous abilities of the nurse as artist. Therefore, important dimensions of the nurse's artistic ability can be seen only when others' responses in the environment are viewed as an integral whole with the nurse's movement.

Movement brings physical and symbolic touch into being. The meaning of touch, considered vitally important in nursing practice, is conveyed through the movement that brings the touch into being and that moves away from the touch. As an example, consider a scene in the movie *Silence Like Glass*, where Eva, a rising star ballerina, faces a devastating malignancy and can no longer dance. Her dance partner, with whom she had dreamed of touring the world, comes to visit. As he is leaving, she reaches out to touch his hand in a loving gesture that also conveys the regret and sorrow of the moment. Ivanoff quickly withdraws his hand from her touch, with a subtle upper body shift backward and a facial expression of repulsion. Here, if we observed just the moment of touch in a snapshot, the meaning of the episode would be lost.

Movement provides a means for a nurse to define the time-space within which care and concern will be expressed (Chinn, Maeve, and Bostick, 1997). As the nurse enters an encounter, body moves, gestures that sometimes include touch, and visual scanning define the space within which the nurse turns attention throughout the encounter. The nurse's moves remain primarily within this space until near the end of the encounter, at which time there occurs a gesture or move, often along with words, that signifies retreat from the encounter.

Movement brings about actions of protection, assistance, comfort, and healing. The intentions that bring these types of moves into being are inherent within the move and serve to define the move. The actual body movement and posturing can be done without intention. With intention, subtleties of posture and sequence of movement can be observed. There is a component of intention that can be sensed, linked to the style of the move, and linked to the physical form and shape of the movement. Moves that mimic those done with intention convey an emptiness and a void that render them technical and mechanical.

Movement is the medium that carries technical skill. Like movement that provides comfort and healing, technical skill performance can be empty and mechanical. What creates an aesthetic performance of a technical skill is the nurse's intention to bring the various elements of the experience and the situation into a coherent, integrated whole, in which all movements fall into right relationship. Being able to do this requires practice (rehearsal) and well-developed skill, but unless the intention is inherent in the performance, the act of doing the technical task remains mechanical. Intention saturates the movements of technical skill with meaning; finely tuned style, timing, finesse, and coordination convey artistic as well as scientific competence.

The five aspects of body-mind-heart movement that contribute to its artistic quality are as follows:

1. Coordinated balance is the concurrent movement of all parts of the body within a whole, smooth, integral pattern. Coordinated balance includes breath patterns as a foundation for the more visible co-ordination of muscle movement. Breath forms the rhythm of the movement and undergirds the movement with strength, both physical and symbolic. Coordinated balance among parts within a sequence of movements requires embodied knowing of the intended flow of the sequence. Cognitive awareness of the flow of sequence of movement can be present, but the more the moves are embodied intelligence and not cognitively processed, the finer and more balanced the coordination.

2. Finesse is the refinement and versatility with which moves are made. Finesse depends on embodied familiarity with the environment, the objects, and the processes with which the nurse works. It reflects integrated knowing of the material world and the capabilities of the body. Finesse comes with practice and experience and can be nurtured with rehearsal, but each individual has different aptitudes for developing finesse with different moves.

3. Style is the unique character that each individual brings to move-ment—the heart of the movement. It is the particular way that a nurse uses movement in the process of bringing intention and action together and the unique artistic expressions that emerge in the creation of an integrated whole. Style can be described and character-ized by the observer, but it cannot be duplicated because it resides as an integral element within the self. There can be no value judgments with respect to style itself, but style is an important aspect that contributes to artistic value. Artistic value resides not in the style per se but in the form of the whole, the meaning that is con-veyed, and the responses that are evoked.

4. Timing involves rhythm, pace, and the placement of various moves with a time sequence of an unfolding experience. The saying that timing is everything certainly applies to the artistic validity of nursing art. Timing is an important factor in narrative interactions as well as movement. Timing is a key marker of intuitive ability, for timing cannot be planned in advance, and it is not cognitively pro-cessed. Rather, timing emerges from apprehension in the mo-ment as an experience unfolds.

5. Synchrony is the ability to bring together elements of the environ-ment, the responses of others, and the situation into an integrated whole. Synchrony depends upon coordination, finesse, style, and timing. It brings all elements of movement together in interaction with the situation.

Movement is a medium that creates the shape of emplotment of the emerging story of lived experience. It is an avenue of communication that shows, demonstrates, opens, assists, and inspires the shift from one moment to the next. When movement is considered as a foundational element of the art of nursing, it acquires symbolic meaning that shapes the form of the whole and the intended feeling response.

The aspects of coordination, finesse, and style can be rehearsed in isolated practice sequences and deliberately planned exercises. Timing and synchrony need to be rehearsed within a situational context because they can be expressed only when situational elements are present. Timing and synchrony can be refined through reflective practice and by placing a situation within a story line to rehearse alternative story lines that incorporate differences of timing and elements of synchrony that might be integrated in a similar but different situation.

Movement exercises, particularly those that are meditative (such as tai chi or yoga), can be used to develop embodied movement skills of coordination, finesse, and style. These forms of movement provide rehearsal in bringing intention and imagery into expression through physical movement. The posturing and movements of these body meditations are consistent with good body mechanics, developing an embodied sense of balance, rhythm, and coordination.

Rehearsal and Engaging a Connoisseur-Critic. Rehearsal can focus on specific aspects of narrative or movement, as suggested in the previous sections. It most often brings several elements together into a situation that is performed either in a protected studio or in a relatively safe actual nursing situation. Engaging a connoisseur-critic to observe the rehearsal is a vital aspect of developing aesthetic ability because developing art form depends on being able to convey a sense of the whole and a sense of feeling. The one who is "performing" cannot be situated in the role of the observer, the audience. Only from the observer's perspective can artistic validity be fully perceived. It is in interaction with the responses of the critic that artists gain insight into the integrity of their expression, deepen their knowledge of their art form, and discover avenues for moving their art to a new realm of possibility (Reed, 1995).

Connoisseur-critics have deep familiarity with and appreciation of the art form. They have developed sufficient skill in the art form to understand the technical expertise that is required. They have studied the theories that pertain to the art form so that they have knowledge of that toward which the art is directed, as well as knowledge of the art form itself. They know the history of the art form and understand how it has changed over time. They are familiar with the cultural context within which the art form is currently placed and the possibilities for new directions that are emerging within the art. Given their expertise, they have developed a keenly trained "eye" and "ear" and "feel" for the art (Chinn, Maeve, and Bostick, 1997). The intention of the connoisseur-critic is to nurture the artist's ability to a new dimension of expression. It is this intention, and its translation into action, that creates a safe environment that nurtures the artist's skill. A skilled teacher is a skilled connoisseur-critic, and a skilled connoisseur-critic is a skilled teacher.

Connoisseurship is integral to the process of developing the art. Skilled critics nurture critical abilities in the novice artist and build the reflective capacities necessary for refining aesthetic ability. Knowledge of the art expands beyond knowing how to place elements into a form. The novice also acquires aesthetic sensitivity to meanings in the art as it is being performed, an educated appreciation of the work of expert practitioners, and openness to inspiration from the work of others.

The primary function of the connoisseur-critic in a rehearsal context is to provide guidance that moves the art form to a new level of development. The critic provides substantive information about aspects of the performance that are well developed and elements of the performance that show promise for development and also specific guidance for taking the performance to a new level of skill. Ideally the critic works with the artist over time so that the critic becomes familiar with the unique abilities and style of the performer and can place each rehearsal in the context of evolving ability. The critic becomes sensitive to signals of emerging ability and moves with the artist to encourage the next move toward artistic competence.

The critic does not give generalized value judgments of "good" or "bad." Value judgments are empty of substantive insight about the performance. The critic does give authentic indicators of the feeling response that the performance elicited, as well as substantive information as to what about the performance elicited response. For example, in response to a nurse's unexpected move that clearly turns an evolving situation in a new direction, the critic might say, "When you did . . . [summarizing the move], at first I felt fearful because it was so unexpected and seemed so daring, so out of place. Then, as soon as I saw what happened next, my heart leaped with joy because clearly you made a breakthrough when you did that." Here, the value-laden responses of fear and joy are grounded in the particular perspective of the critic and explicitly linked with the nurse's actions.

When the critic observes something that could change or that needs to change, rather than render a value judgment of "bad," the critic gives specific guidance for the next step and, if possible, places the element within the context of the performer's history. For example, in response to a move that is awkward and poorly timed, the critic's response might be: "I sensed that you were distracted and tense today when you . . . [summarizing the move]. One thing that you might try next time is to pause and breathe for a moment before you jump into this kind of challenge. Spend a moment getting clear about your intentions as you gather your equipment, and breathe!" Or the critic might respond, "You lacked finesse when you were . . . [summarizing the incident]. Here is a small sequence of moves that you can practice over the next week that I think will help. Start out slowly, and practice breathing and establishing a rhythm, a flow."

Connoisseurship implies a creativity of its own in that the critic engages in observing the rehearsal with a sense of openness to insights that have not previously been conceived. It also implies a discipline in that the critic offers a trained perspective and expectation concerning artistic validity. The elements that the critic observes in light of expectations for artistic validity include the following:

- *Voice intonation and expression in narrative.* The way that narrative is delivered carries the feeling of the narrative. The critic notices the feeling that is elicited from the narrative and notes specific elements of expression that appear associated with the response.
- *Substance of the narrative interactions.* The critic notices words, phrases, and narrative sequences and how they are framed within the whole.
- *Synchrony of movement.* The critic observes how movement is situated within the context of the situation and provides guidance for developing skill in areas that interfere with integrity and synchrony.
- *Synchrony between movement and narrative.* The critic observes the ways in which movement and words come together to form a whole within the interaction and ways in which movement and narrative fall into place in right relationship.
- *Perceived intention and emotion.* The critic senses the intention that is communicated by the nurse, which may not coincide with the nurse's felt intention. When the perceived (received) intention and the nurse's felt intention do not coincide, elements of artistic form might need to shift to adequately convey the felt intention.
- *Synchrony of interaction.* The critic notices the responses of others in the situation and the rhythm and flow in the interactions, which reveal possible avenues for developing the art.

AESTHETIC KNOWLEDGE FORMS: CRITICISM AND WORKS OF ART

Works of art that are developed to show and symbolize artistic qualities that are expressed in nursing practice are the nondiscursive form of aesthetic knowledge. Works of art can take the form of visual paintings, drawings, or photographs; literary works such as poetry and fiction; dance; music; or any other art form. Works of art express meanings in the nursing experience as the artist perceives them; they are expressed in the unique expression of the artist. Those who see or hear or read what is expressed in a work of art also engage in an aesthetic experience of perceiving meaning in a situation, often meaning that would not otherwise be perceived, except for the experience of engaging in the art form as observer.

Aesthetic criticism is the formal discursive form of expression of aesthetic knowledge. Aesthetic criticism can focus on the art that is expressed in nursing practice or on a formally developed work of art inspired from nursing experience. Aesthetic criticism gives insight into the art form, interprets the work of selected artists, and deepens appreciation of the art. It is constructed from the work of the connoisseur-critic, who selects the work of one or more artists as a point of focus. The critic engages in deep reflection into the meanings of the art and the technical adequacy of the art, systematically explores the significance of one or more interpretations of the art, and places the art in a historical and cultural context.

Aesthetic criticism includes the following essential elements (Chinn, Maeve, and Bostick, 1997):

- *Historical integration.* Historical integration is done on two levels: the history of the art as an art form and the personal artistic history of the artist. The significance of an artist's work can be interpreted only in light of that which has come before. The critic examines evidence of change and continuity in the artist's own history and interprets the meanings of each of these threads. The critic also presents threads of change and continuity in the art form and places this artist's work within the context of those threads. Johnson's (1994) philosophic analysis of literature concerning the art of nursing, while explicitly not an historical study, provides evidence of past conceptualizations of the art of nursing and identifies certain consistencies that have appeared within the literature over time. The aesthetic critic would draw on this and other sources to use as a mirror from which to reflect the meaning of the work that is the focus of the criticism.
- *Comparative description of the art form.* The critic examines the form that this artist takes in the artistic process and compares this artist's work with that of known forms of the art. By drawing comparisons, the critic substantiates the unique aspects of this artist's work and the significance of this artist's work for the discipline.
- *Consideration of plausible interpretations of meaning.* The critic transfers stance among a number of plausible interpretive meanings of the art and explores what the various meanings contribute to aesthetic understanding in the discipline. The critic may develop a preferred interpretation, but the stance remains open and fluid.
- *Translation of future possibility.* The critic explores the directions that this artist might take and what the work of this artist contributes to the future development of the discipline. This aspect of criticism sets the stage for inspiration—for the artist and for others in the discipline.

PROCESSES FOR AFFIRMING AESTHETIC KNOWLEDGE: APPRECIATION AND INSPIRATION

As with the other patterns of knowing, for knowledge to become meaningful within the discipline, members of the discipline engage in collective processes to affirm what is valuable for the discipline. In the sphere of aesthetics, collective affirmation of aesthetic knowledge involves appreciation and inspiration. There are three guiding principles upon which appreciation and inspiration are founded: (1) unique, creative expression grounded in the immediacy and enduring wholeness of human experience, (2) expanded dimensions of plausible meanings, and (3) illuminated possibilities for the future.

Shared works of art set before the discipline representations that are unique in temporal time and space but that are grounded in the wholeness of human experience. Aesthetic criticism reveals the particular uniqueness by highlighting and bringing to conscious awareness aspects of creativity that may not be readily perceptible to the casual observer. Unique features serve to distinguish this work from any other and reveal possibilities in human experience and expression that have not existed before and will not be replicated. At the same time valued works of art touch chords of immediacy and call forth human responses in the moment. The capacity to call forth human response in the moment reflects the art's power to reflect enduring wholeness—that which is shared and common in the human experience.

Valued works of art, because of their uniqueness and their ability to call forth human response, offer to the culture expanded dimensions of meaning. Aesthetic criticism explores various dimensions of meaning that are conveyed through the art and offers plausible interpretations of the meanings. The response that is elicited by the art deepens the observer-participant's appreciation of experience and meaning to an extent that would not otherwise be possible.

Valued works of art inspire new and different directions for the future. Aesthetic criticism articulates possible directions, but any observer-participant can also find inspiration within the aesthetic experience. Other artists gain inspiration for their own work by deepening their appreciation of the valued art. The observer-participant gains inspiration relative to life experience; new possibilities, new directions, and different paths to travel enter the imagination and become seeds of possibility.

CONCLUSION

In this chapter we have reviewed meanings of art and aesthetics in nursing and presented methods for developing aesthetic knowing and knowledge in nursing. Aesthetics presents unique challenges that bring concerns of being (ontology) and knowing (epistemology) together and can open doors for the experience of the whole.

Reference List

Benner PA, Tanner CA, Chesla CA: *Expertise in nursing practice: caring, clinical judgment, and ethics,* New York, 1996, Springer.

Benner P, Wrubel J: *The primacy of caring: stress and coping in health and illness,* Menlo Park, Calif, 1989, Addison Wesley.

Carper BA: Fundamental patterns of knowing in nursing, *Adv Nurs Sci* 1:13, 1978.

Chinn PL: Developing a method for aesthetic knowing in nursing. In Chinn PL, Watson J, editors: *Art and aesthetics in nursing,* New York, 1994, National League for Nursing Press.

Chinn PL, Maeve MK, Bostick C: Aesthetic inquiry and the art of nursing, *Sch Inq Nurs Pract* 11:83, 1997.

Chinn PL, Watson J: *Art & aesthetics in nursing,* New York, 1994, National League for Nursing Press.

Eisner E: Aesthetic modes of knowing. In Eisner E, editor: *Learning and teaching the ways of knowing: part II,* Chicago, 1985, University of Chicago Press.

Johnson JL: A dialectical examination of nursing art, *Adv Nurs Sci* 17:1, 1994.

Johnson JL: Dialectical analysis concerning the rational aspect of the art of nursing, *Image J Nurs Sch* 28:169, 1996.

Maeve MK: Coming to moral consciousness through the art of nursing narratives. In Chinn PL, Watson J, editors: *Art and aesthetics in nursing,* New York, 1994, National League for Nursing Press.

Mattingly C: The narrative nature of clinical reasoning. In Mattingly C, Fleming MH, editors: *Clinical reasoning: forms of inquiry in a therapeutic practice,* Philadelphia, 1994, FA Davis.

Mattingly C, Fleming MH: *Clinical reasoning: forms of inquiry in a therapeutic practice,* Philadelphia, 1994, FA Davis.

Oettinger KB: Toward inner freedom, *Am J Nurs* 39:1224, 1939.

Reed PG: A treatise on nursing knowledge development for the 21st century: beyond postmodernism, *Adv Nurs Sci* 17:70, 1995.

Sandelowski M: On the aesthetics of qualitative research, *Image J Nurs Sch* 27:205, 1995.

Silva MC, Sorrell JM, Sorrell CD: From Carper's patterns of knowing to ways of being: an ontological philosophical shift in nursing, *Adv Nurs Sci* 18:1, 1995.

Sorrell JM: Remembrance of things past through writing: esthetic patterns of knowing in nursing, *Adv Nurs Sci* 17:60, 1994.

Vezeau TM: Narrative inquiry in nursing. In Chinn PL, Watson J, editors: *Art and aesthetics in nursing,* New York, 1994, National League for Nursing Press.

Epilogue: A Note on Praxis

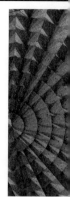

Of old the nursing sisters of the religious orders, closely confined in shackles of mental subjugation and social renunciation, consciously withdrew from all participation in things of the world . . . held no radical hopes of remaking the social order about them. . . . If their paths were strewn with the wrecks of social justice they patiently and untiringly bound up the wounds and nursed the victims without a protest. We have cast off their shackles because we refuse to be cut off from the world about us . . . human society can be voluntarily and consciously built into nobler and fairer forms than those of the past. (p. 896)

Lavinia L. Dock (1907)

As we come to the end of this phase of our work, it seems important to reflect on our intentions and hopes for this major revision. We have introduced into this edition the concept of praxis, and now at the conclusion of the text we wish to focus clearly on the ideas represented by this work and why it is so central to our motives and our efforts to provide this integrated approach to knowledge development.

Praxis is a word that is very much alive in the nursing literature today. Originally the meaning of praxis was closely linked to practice or "to do." Today, when we use the word *praxis,* it carries connotations that are different from practice in the usual sense. The word now is closely linked to critical social theory and means acting with awareness, a simultaneous doing while reflecting on the doing, always shifting what is done, based on insights from reflection.

The use of any word implies its social value. A word communicates something that is necessary. By embracing the word *praxis,* we acknowledge that the word *practice* is no longer adequate to represent the ideal of nursing.

In our view *practice* has the connotation of replication or duplication of the status quo. Research and theory development, processes that are closely linked with science, also have this connotation. *Research,* as Wilma Scott Heide (1985) astutely noted, often means search over and over again for the same old thing. She advocated shifting to future search, with the intention to create something new.

Theory created out of research is often represented as the template we can overlay on practice to enable us, subsequently, to explain and predict what will happen. Looking back at history can show us important lessons and assure that we do not re-create a past that needs to change. The important shift to create a desired future is to reflect critically on what has come before, to use our creative powers to imagine something new, and to act to begin to create that which better serves us in the future.

We defined *praxis* as thoughtful reflection and action that occur in synchrony. Praxis is prospective. It creates a desired future. Praxis is value-grounded action that integrates ontology and epistemology; praxis integrates who we are and what we know. If we are serious about praxis, we must change our approach to knowledge generation. Our personal seriousness about the concept of praxis brought us to the position that we could no longer write a book that dealt only with empiric theory. We could not write a book that focused on the activities of knowledge development without showing how knowledge and knowing come together, how what nurses do in practice is integrally a part of both knowing and knowledge, and vice versa. Praxis at the core of our thinking put praxis at the core of our model.

The central core of the model we introduced in Chapter 1 represents this core of praxis. The core includes scientific competence, moral-ethical comportment, therapeutic use of self, and transformative art-acts. Although each pattern has an expression of knowing associated with it, the central core is most appropriately thought of as an ontologic expression of knowing and knowledge—that is, ways of being-doing in relation to what is known. Although the central expressions of knowing are grounded in the individual knowledge expressions related to each pattern, they are never fully expressed as knowledge but as integrated knowing-being. What we are trying to depict is knowing as being and being as knowing. In the central core, ontology and epistemology blend, which is exactly what is required for praxis. We realize that pulling out expressions of integrated knowing-being is a move destined to bring criticism. Yet we think it is important to understanding. Trying to create understandable language and visual expressions of these complex ideas is an ongoing challenge that, we think, would defy anyone's creativity.

Praxis implies the creation and shaping of the future. Praxis requires a vision of the future we want to create. The vision is not confined to any one pattern but is rather reflected in all knowing patterns. Aesthetic knowledge, personal knowledge, scientific knowledge, and ethical knowledge reflect in various ways the collective vision to be scrutinized and inspected. Knowledge, as much as it might embody appropriate values for nursing, is not enough. Critical thinking is not enough, and thoughtful reflection is not enough. Praxis brings all of these aspects together to form a whole.

Praxis requires action that is motivated by values that are constantly questioned and fully understood to be reflective of political agendas that may not favor their implementation. In our model we have depicted ways whereby the actions that embody our knowledge are questioned and understood. The political realities of change, the devaluing of much of what nursing represents, and the global status of women for a profession dominated by women must be understood—really understood—if praxis is to occur. We believe our model moves us in that direction. The questions we have posed in relation to each knowing pattern do not focus on that pattern alone but require us to look at the whole of knowing-being in nursing. When you ask, Do I know what I do? Do I do what I know? therapeutic use of self alone is not questioned. Rather the question addresses how individual personhood influences—indeed, how it creates—integrated scientific competence, moral-ethical comportment, therapeutic use of self, and transformative art-acts. Praxis requires a dialectic, a communication between the old notions of "research, theory, and practice." It requires communication between "the academics and the practitioners." It requires so powerful a connection that these distinctions will no longer make sense and be lost from our language.

What motivates this epilogue is a need to share our commitments and hopes for what we might collectively accomplish with a focus on knowing and knowledge. One of the highest honors we know is for you to take our ideas, make them your own, develop and use them, and share your insights with the nursing community. This can happen only if our ideas are communicated, and this is what we have done.

This book is not a finished work and never will be. Ever since Carper's original work appeared in the premiere issue of *Advances in Nursing Science*, we have been thinking about, developing, and working with these fundamental knowing patterns. Carper's work was extremely useful and important for us because it named and made room for much of what we knew was important in nursing. In our earlier careers we found ourselves "squeezing" other patterns of knowing and being into the inappropriate frame of empirics because other patterns of knowing had not been named. In many ways Carper's work provided tangible roots for our ideas. Carper's work also helped to establish a meaningful connection with many nurses who had gone before. We hope our work may do the same for you.

So, as we close this chapter of our labor of love, these are our commitments, our hopes, and our intentions. We view it as a beginning. These are ways of being that we intend to keep in the forefront. This book has been exciting work for us. We invite you to share in the journey that will take us to a new future that is grounded in values that represent the very best that nursing can be.

Reference List

Dock L: Some urgent social claims, *Am J Nurs* 7:895, 1907.
Heide WS: *Feminism for the health of it,* Buffalo, 1985, Margaretdaughters.

Appendix A

Interpretive Summary: Examples of Broad Theoretic Frameworks Defining the Scope, Philosophy, and General Characteristics of Nursing

The summaries provided here include published writings prior to 1991. The summaries are not complete descriptions or critical reflections of the theorists' works. Rather they are interpretive descriptions of essential features of selected conceptual frameworks for illustrative purposes. A notation of the theoretic writing that we used in preparing the summary precedes the summary. The original terminology of the theorists has been retained.

H. E. PEPLAU

Interpersonal relations in nursing, 1952
The art and science of nursing, 1988

The patient is an individual with a felt need, and nursing is a process that is both interpersonal and therapeutic. Nursing is the simultaneous application of art and science. The overall goal or purpose of nursing is to educate and be a maturing force so that personality development (a new view of self) occurs. This purpose is achieved when the nurse, as a medium for change, enters into a personal relationship with an individual, the patient, when a felt need presents itself. The personal relationship in nursing provides for meeting the individual patient's needs and assists the two persons (nurse and patient) with different goals to develop or assume congruent goals. The nurse-patient relationship occurs in phases, during which the nurse functions as a resource person, a counselor, and a surrogate. There are four phases: orientation, identification, exploitation, and resolution. When a person with a need seeks help, the nurse assists in orientation to the problem. During phase 1 the illness event is integrated. The person learns the facets of the difficulty and the extent of need for help. Orientating to use of services, productively exploiting anxiety and tension, and learning the limits of necessary space and freedom also occur. This helps to ensure that the illness event is not repressed. When orientation is completed to a given degree, the phase of identification begins. In phase 2 the patient assumes a posture of interdependence, dependence, or independence in relation to the nurse. The nurse assists the patient during this phase by taking into consideration the services needed and the patient's history. Identification helps assure the patient that the nurse can understand the interpersonal meaning of the patient's situation. When identification is accomplished, phase 3, exploitation, begins. In this phase, the patient derives full value from the relationship by using the services available on the basis of self-interest and needs. Resolution, the final phase, occurs as old needs are met. With resolution of older needs, newer and more mature needs emerge. When needs are resolved, the person is freed from dependence on others. The maturing force of nursing is realized as the personality develops through the educational, therapeutic, and interpersonal process of nursing. The phases of the relationship are serial, and the patient assumes an active role.

During the dyadic nurse-patient relationship and the more extensive nursing relationships with communities, nurses assume many roles, including stranger, teacher, resource person, surrogate, leader, and counselor. Multiple roles occur as a result of multiple client problems and needs in individual interpersonal relationships, team functions, and varying social and professional expectations. The overall goal for professional nursing is the same as for the nurse-patient dyads: to implement a process that facilitates personality development by helping people use forces and experiences to ensure maximum productivity.

F. G. ABDELLAH, I. L. BELAND, A. MARTIN, AND R. V. MATHENEY

Patient-centered approaches to nursing, 1960

The patient or family presents with nursing problems that the nurse helps them address through her professional function. The nurse addresses 21 problem categories: (1) hygiene and physical comfort, (2) activity and rest, (3) safety, (4) body mechanics, (5) oxygenation, (6) nutrition, (7) elimination, (8) fluid and electrolytes, (9) responses to disease, (10) regulatory mechanisms, (11) sensory function, (12) feelings and reactions, (13) emotions and illness interrelationships, (14) communication, (15) interpersonal relationships, (16) spirituality, (17) therapeutic environment, (18) awareness of self, (19) limitation acceptance, (20) resources to resolve problems, and (21) role of social problems in illness.

Nursing problems are both overt or obvious and covert. Nurses must be aware of covert problems to meet care requirements. Overt and covert problems must be identified to make a nursing diagnosis. Identification of problems precedes solution. The nursing process is the method nurses use to establish and focus on a nursing diagnosis. The overall goal is a client's fullest possible functioning.

Individualized patient care is important for nursing. Both patients and nurses should be aware of the wholeness of clients and the need for continuity of care from before hospitalization to afterward. Individualized care will require changes in the organization and administration of nursing services and education.

I. J. ORLANDO

The dynamic nurse-patient relationship:
function, process and principles, 1961
The discipline and teaching of nursing process: an evaluation study, 1972

The patient is an individual with a need that, if supplied, diminishes distress, increases adequacy, or enhances well-being. Needs include requirements for implementing physicians' plans or other innate requirements. The nurse acts to meet needs and thus alleviate distress.

Patients with needs behave verbally and nonverbally in a given manner. The nurse reacts to patient behavior by ascertaining both the meaning of the distress and what would alleviate the distress. Finally the nurse acts to alleviate the distress. Distress can be due to (1) physical limitations, either temporary or permanent; (2) adverse reactions to the setting, such as being misinterpreted or misinterpreting; and (3) inability to communicate.

Three elements—patient behavior, nurse reactions, and nurse actions—compose a nursing situation. Patient behavior and nurse reactions relate to the assessment phase of the nursing process and involve ongoing interaction with the nurse. Having clearly ascertained the need through assessment, the nurse acts automatically or deliberatively. Automatic actions are those carried out for reasons other than resolving an immediate need, whereas deliberative actions seek to meet assessed needs. Automatic actions make problems by creating situational conflict that is evidenced through lack of resolution of needs and cooperation (i.e., distress is not alleviated).

Deliberative action yields solutions to problems and also prevents problems. Once the nursing action occurs, the nurse evaluates patient behavior to determine if the need has been met and resultant distress has been alleviated. The overall goal is to meet needs and, in that way, to alleviate distress.

E. WIEDENBACH

Clinical nursing: a helping art, 1964

The patient is an individual under treatment or care who experiences needs. Needs are requirements for maintenance or stability in a situation that may be perceived by the individual as a requirement for help and may be met by the person or others. Also, people may have needs and not seek help or may help themselves without recognizing a need. Needs for help are defined as "measures or actions required and desired, which potentially restore or extend ability to cope with situational demands" (p. 6). Nursing is concerned with patients' needs for help. What the nurse does and how she or he does it compose clinical nursing. Clinical nursing has four components: (1) philosophy, (2) purpose, (3) practice, and (4) art.

Philosophy is a personal stance of the nurse that embodies attitudes toward reality, and purpose is the overall goal. The purpose of clinical nursing is "to facilitate efforts of individuals to overcome obstacles which interfere with abilities to respond capably to demands made by the condition, environment, situation or time" (p. 15). This purpose is the embodiment of meeting needs for help, which implies goal-directed, deliberate, patient-centered practice actions that require (1) knowledge (factual, speculative, and practical), (2) judgment, and (3) skills (procedural and communication). Practice includes four components: (1) identification of the perceived need for help, (2) ministration of help needed, (3) validation that help given was the help needed, and (4) coordination of help and resources for help (i.e., reporting, consulting, and conferring). The art of clinical nursing requires individualized interpretations of behavior in meeting needs for help.

The helping process is triggered by patient behavior that the nurse perceives and interprets. In interpreting behavior the nurse compares the perception to an expectation or hope. Nursing actions may be rational, reactionary, and deliberative. A rational response by the nurse is based on the immediate perception without going beyond to explore hidden meaning. A reactionary response is taken in reaction to strong feelings. Deliberative actions—the desirable mode—intelligibly fulfill nursing's purpose. Identification of needs for help involves (1) observing inconsistencies, acquiring information about how patients mean the cue given, or determining the basis for an observed inconsistency; (2) determining the cause of the discomfort or need for help; and (3) determining whether the need for help can be met by the patient or whether assistance is required. Once needs for help are identified, ministration and validation that help was given follow.

The practice of clinical nursing is bounded by professional, local, legal, and personal constraints. Clinical nursing practice is supported by nursing administration, nursing education, nursing organizations, and nursing research. The clinical goal is to meet needs for help, integrating the practice and process of nursing. Greater professional goals include conservation of life and promotion of health.

L. E. HALL

Another view of nursing care and quality, 1966

The patient is a unity composed of three overlapping parts: a person (the core aspect), a pathology and treatment (the cure aspect), and a body (the care aspect). The nurse is a bodily caregiver. Provision of bodily care allows the nurse to comfort and learn the patient's pathology, treatment aspect, and person. Understanding, resulting from the integration of all three areas, allows the nurse to be an effective teacher and nurturer. The patient learns and is nurtured in the person (that is, in the core aspect). Nurturance leads to effective rehabilitation, greater levels of self-actualization, and self-love.

Nursing occurs during one of two phases of medical care. Phase 1 medical care is the diagnostic and treatment phase; phase 2 is the evaluative, follow-up phase. The professional nurse's role is in phase 2, and professional nursing practice requires a setting in which patients are free to learn. In phase 2 the nurse's goal is to help the patient learn. Motivation to learn is assured by advocating the patient's learning goals and not the doctor's curative goals. Once patient learning goals are codetermined with the nurse and motivation therefore assured, the patient will learn, and nurturance, rehabilitation, and self-love follow. The overall goal for the client is rehabilitation, which inspires a greater measure of self-actualization and self-love.

V. HENDERSON

The nature of nursing, 1966

The patient is an individual who requires help toward independence. The nurse assists the individual, whether ill or not, to perform activities that will contribute to health, recovery, or peaceful death—activities that the individual who had necessary strength, will, or knowledge would perform unaided. The process of nursing strives to do this as rapidly as possible, and the goal is independence. The nurse manages this process independently of physicians. Help toward independence is given autonomously by the nurse in relation to (1) breathing, (2) eating and drinking, (3) elimination, (4) movement and posture, (5) sleep and rest, (6) clothing, (7) maintenance of body temperature, (8) cleaning and grooming of the body and integument protection, (9) avoidance of environmental dangers and injury of others, (10) communication, (11) worship, (12) work, (13) play and participation in recreation, and (14) learning and discovery. Nursing can be evaluated as a profession on the basis of the extent to which it enables the individual to achieve each of these functions autonomously.

The role and functions of professional nursing vary with the situation. If the total health care team comprises a pie graph in health care situations, in some situations no role exists for certain health care workers. Although there is always a role for family and patients, the pie wedges for team members vary in size according to (1) the problem of the patient, (2) the patient's self-help ability, and (3) the help resources. Central to nursing that seeks to help patients toward independence is empathetic understanding and unlimited knowledge. Empathetic understanding grounded in genuine interest will lead to helping the family understand what a patient needs. The ultimate goal for the nurse is to practice autonomously in helping patients who lack knowledge, physical strength, or strength of will in growth toward independence. Because of this function, nurses seek and promote research, education, and work settings that facilitate this goal.

J. TRAVELBEE

Interpersonal aspects of nursing, 1966, 1971

Nursing is an interpersonal process aimed at assisting individuals, families, or communities to prevent or cope with the process of illness and suffering and, if necessary, to find meaning in the experience. Nursing's purpose is achieved through human-to-human relationships, which are established by a disciplined intellectual approach to problems, combined with therapeutic use of self. Human-to-human relationships require transcending roles of nurse and patient to establish relatedness and rapport and respond to the humanness of others. Nursing activities are a means to establishing relatedness and rapport and achieving nursing's purpose. Nurses' values and beliefs determine the quality of nursing care provided and thus the extent to which nurses are able to help the ill find meaning in their situation.

Illness and suffering are spiritual, emotional, and physical experiences. The nurse assists the ill patient to experience hope as a means of coping with illness and suffering. Communication, a central concept for Travelbee, implies guiding, planning, and purposely directing interaction to fulfill nursing's purpose. Communication is instrumental in establishing related-ness and rapport (knowing persons), ascertaining and meeting nursing needs, and fulfilling nursing's purpose. Communication also implies that exchanged messages are understood. Communication techniques should enable the nurse to explore and understand the meaning of the person's communication. Establishment of the human-to-human relationship is phasic. The phases are (1) the original encounter, (2) emerging identities, (3) empathy, and (4) sympathy (1971, p. 119). In such a relationship the needs of the person are met. Achievement of a human-to-human relation-ship requires openness to experiences and freedom to use personal and experiential background to appreciate and understand the experiences of others.

Health and illness may be defined subjectively and objectively. Objective criteria depend on cultural and societal norms, whereas subjective criteria are peculiar to the human being. The meaning of the symptoms of illness (or criteria for health) for the person is more significant than affixing a label of health or illness to its results.

M. E. LEVINE

The four conservation principles of nursing, 1967
Introduction to clinical nursing, 1973
The conservation principles: twenty years later, 1989

A person is a wholistic being whose open and fluid boundaries coexist with the environment, which may be perceptual, operational, and conceptual, and is a unity who is to remain conserved and integral. He or she sends messages that reflect his or her current adaptive state. Adaptation is a method of change, and change is life process. When adaptation fails, conservation is threatened, and adaptation needs occur. Adaptive needs are reflected in messages sent.

Nursing occurs at the interface between the open and fluid boundaries of whole persons and environments. The nurse receives and interprets messages and intervenes supportively or therapeutically. Intervention is guided by the four principles of conservation: conservation of energy, structural integrity, personal integrity, and social integrity. Conservation, based on an assessment of a person's adaptive needs, aids adaptation. When a patient's energy and structural, personal, and social integrity are conserved—that is, when the nurse acts therapeutically—adaptation can better occur, and the person achieves a state of unity and integrity. When conservation cannot be effected in the face of overwhelming adaptation needs, death ensues. Supportive interventions, such as assisting a client toward peaceful death, are appropriate when adaptation is failing without hope of reversal. The goal for nursing is the wholeness of the patient, brought about by conservation in the four areas when adaptive needs are manifested.

M. E. ROGERS

An introduction to the theoretical basis of nursing, 1970
Nursing: a science of unitary man, 1980
Science of unitary human beings: a paradigm for nursing, 1983
Nursing: a science of unitary human beings, 1989

A unitary human being is an energy field coextensive with the universe. Human-environment boundaries are only conceptually imposed and are arbitrary. The unity of human beings and environment is plausible, considering the sameness of matter and energy. Humans are more than and different from the sum of their parts, and generalities about the whole cannot be made from a study of the parts. The energy composing unitary human beings and the environmental field is characterized by four dimensions, in which a given point in time is not tenable. The four concepts—energy fields, openness, pattern and organization, and four-dimensionality—are used to derive principles that postulate how human beings develop. These principles are (1) integrality (formerly complimentarity), (2) resonancy, and (3) helicy. According to the principle of integrality, the human and environmental fields interact mutually and simultaneously. Resonancy postulates the nature of wave pattern changes as continuous from lower-frequency to higher-frequency patterns. Helicy asserts that field changes are innovative, probabilistic, and characterized by increasing diversity of field patterns.

Nursing seeks to care for unitary human beings in accordance with its science and art. Science is emergent and based on research and logical analysis of the principles of homeodynamics. Nursing science seeks to describe, explain, and predict. Art is the imaginative and creative use of knowledge and science. Nursing's goal is maximization of health potentials of individuals, family, and groups consistent with health's ever-changing nature. It is achieved by artfully applying emerging science, based on the principles of homeodynamics.

D. E. OREM

Nursing: concepts of practice, 1971, 1980, 1985, 1991

Orem's self-care deficit theory of nursing includes theories of (1) self-care deficit, (2) self-care, and (3) nursing system. Self-care deficit theory postulates that people benefit from nursing in that they have health-related limitations in providing self-care. Self-care theory postulates that self-care and care of dependents are learned behaviors that purposely regulate human structural integrity, functioning, and development. Nursing systems theory postulates that nursing systems form when nurses prescribe, design, and provide nursing that regulates the individual's self-care capabilities and meets therapeutic self-care requirements.

Assumptions basic to the general theory are as follows:

1. Humans require deliberate input to self and environment to be alive and to function.
2. The power to act deliberately is exercised in caring for self and others.
3. Mature humans sometimes experience limitations in their ability to care for self and others.
4. Humans discover, develop, and transmit ways to care for self and others.
5. Humans structure relationships and tasks to provide self-care.

Humans need continuous self-care maintenance and regulation and provide this by caring for self, which enables purposeful action. Self-care activities maintain life, health, and well-being. Health refers to the state of a person, which is characterized by soundness or wholeness of developed human structures and bodily and mental functioning. Well-being refers to a person's perceived condition of existence, which is characterized by experiences of contentment, pleasure, happiness, movement toward self-ideals, and continuing personalization.

Three kinds of self-care requisites are universal, developmental, and health deviation. Universal requirements relate to meeting common human needs. Developmental self-care requisites relate to conditions that promote developmental processes throughout the life cycle. Health deviation self-care requisites relate to self-care that prevents defects and deviations from normal structure and integrity and those that control the extension and effects of such defects.

Adults care for themselves, whereas infants, the aged, the ill, and the disabled require assistance with self-care activities. When self-care action is limited because of the health state or needs of the care recipient, nursing responds and provides a legitimate service. Thus patients are people with health-related self-care deficits. Two variables affect these deficits: self-care agency (ability) and self-care demands.

Self-care agency is a learned ability and is deliberate action. Given their focus on care of patients with health-related limitations in self-care abilities, nurses must accurately diagnose self-care agency. Thus they must have information about deficits and their reasons for existing. Such information is basic to selecting helping methods.

Nursing agency regulates or develops patient's self-care agency and ability to meet therapeutic self-care demand. Nursing is a helping service that involves acting or doing for another, guiding and supporting another, providing a developmental environment, and teaching another. Nursing agency varies with educational preparation, orientation to practice situations, mastery of technologies of practice, and ability to accept, work with, and care for others.

Nursing systems may be wholly compensatory, partially compensatory, or supportive-educative. Wholly compensatory systems are required for patients unable to monitor their environment and process information. Such patients are unable to control their movement and position and are unresponsive to stimuli. Partially compensatory systems are designed for patients with limitations in movement as a result of pathology or injury or who are under medical orders to restrict their movements. Supportive-educative systems are designed for patients who need to learn to perform self-care measures and need assistance to do so. Nursing systems are formed to regulate self-care capabilities and meet therapeutic self-care requirements.

I. M. KING

Toward a theory for nursing: general concepts of human behavior, 1971
A theory for nursing: systems, concepts, process, 1981
King's general systems framework and theory, 1989

The patient is a personal system within the environment who coexists with other personal systems. Individuals form groups that comprise interpersonal systems, and interpersonal systems contribute to social systems. Thus patient and nurse are composed of personal systems as subsystems within interpersonal and social systems. The nurse must understand given aspects of all three systems. Concepts identified for each system affect total system function. There are three comprehensive concepts: perception for the personal system, organization for the social system, and interaction for the interpersonal system. Personal system concepts related to perception include self, body image, growth and development, time, space, and learning. The nurse also must have knowledge of role, communication, transaction, and stress to understand interactions central to interpersonal system function. Because interaction occurs within social systems—including family, belief, educational, and work systems—nurses require knowledge or organizational concepts of power, authority, control, status, and decision making to function adequately.

The focus for nursing is the human being in the system context. The goal is health. Health implies helping people in groups attain, maintain, and restore health; live with chronic illness or disability; or die with dignity. Interactions of the individual with the environment are significant in influencing life and health. Nurse and patient meet in a health care organization—a patient who needs help and a nurse who offers help. Nurse and patient perceive one another, act and react, interact, and transact. In this process, presenting conditions are recognized, goal-related decisions are made, and motivation to exert control over events to achieve goals occurs. Transactions are basic to goal attainment and include social exchange, bargaining and negotiating, and sharing a frame of reference toward mutual goal setting. Transactions require perceptual accuracy in nurse-client interactions and congruence between role performance and role expectation for nurse and client. Transactions lead to goal attainment, satisfaction, effective care, and enhanced growth and development. The goal of nursing process interaction is transaction, which leads to attainment of goals set in relation to health promotion, maintenance, and recovery from illness.

B. NEUMAN

The Betty Neuman health care systems model:
a total person approach to patient problems, 1980
The Neuman systems model, 1982, 1989

The person is a unique, wholistic system yet possesses a common range of normal characteristics and responses. Persons are a dynamic composite of physiologic, psychologic, sociocultural, developmental, and spiritual variables. These variables interact with internal and external environmental stressors. The wholistic system of the person is open. As an open system it interacts with, adjusts to, and is adjusted by the environment. The external environment is defined as all that interfaces with the person's system. The internal and external environments are a source of stressors that have different potentials to disturb the normal line of defense and disrupt the system. The normal line of defense is essentially the usual steady state of the individual and is composed of the normal range of responses to stressors within people that evolve over time. The flexible line of defense cushions and protects individuals from stressors. Lines of resistance are conceptualized as internal factors that help people defend against stressors, and they protect the core structure and stabilize and return individuals to a normal line of defense when stressors break through.

The system's model is based on an individual's relationship to stress, reaction to it, and reconstitution factors that are dynamic in nature. The nurse assesses, manages, and evaluates patient systems. Nursing's focus is the variables that affect a person's response to stressors. Assessment of individuals considers knowledge of factors influencing a patient's perceptual field, the meaning stressors have to a patient as validated by patient and caregiver, and factors the caregiver believes influence the patient situation. Basically, nursing focuses on the occurrence of stressors, the organism's response to them, and the state of the organism. Primary prevention identifies and allays risk factors associated with stressors; it focuses on protecting the normal line of defense and strengthening the flexible line of defense. Secondary prevention is related to symptomatology, intervention priorities, and treatment; it helps to strengthen internal lines of defense. Death occurs if the basic core structure of the system fails to support the intervention. Tertiary prevention protects reconstitution or return to wellness following treatment.

Nursing acts to impede or arrest an entropic state or a state of disorder and disorganization. Health is a state of movement toward negentropy or evolution; it is a state of inertness free from disrupting needs. Health implies a homeostatic balance. This balance depends on free energy flow between the organism and the environment. In health the system's normal line of defense is maintained, and the lines of resistance are intact; the basic structural elements of the system are preserved.

C. ROY

Introduction to nursing: an adaptation model, 1976, 1984
The Roy adaptation model, 1980, 1989
Theory construction in nursing: an adaptation model, 1981
(with S. Roberts)

The person is an adaptive system. System inputs include (1) three classes of stimuli (focal, contextual, residual) that arise from within the person and the external environment and (2) the adaptation level. Adaptation level is fluid, is composed of all three classes of stimuli, and represents the person's standard or range of stimuli in which responses will be adaptive.

Inputs are mediated by the control process subsystems of cognate and regulator coping mechanisms. The regulator mechanism is an automatic neuroendocrine response, whereas the cognator subsystems represent perception, information processing, and judgments influenced by learning and emotions. Coping activity may or may not be adequate to maintain integrity. A system difficulty is present when coping activity is inadequate as a result of need excesses or deficits.

The system effectors are the adaptive modes. These modes (physiologic, self-concept, role function, and interdependence) are the form in which regulator and cognator subsystems manifest their activity.

The adaptive system (person's) output is a response that may be adaptive or ineffective. Adaptive responses are those that contribute to adaptation goals (i.e., responses that promote growth, survival, reproduction, and self-mastery). Adaptation is an ongoing purposive response. Adaptive responses contribute to health and the process of being and becoming integrated; ineffective responses do not.

Using nursing process, the nurse promotes adaptive responses in the adaptive modes during health and illness. Thus energy is freed from inadequate coping to promote health and wellness. System responses in each mode are assessed (i.e., described according to objective and subjective data; first-level assessment). Behaviors can be assessed by observation, measurement, and interviews. A tentative judgment about whether the behavior is adaptive or ineffective is then made, and stimuli influencing the adaptive system are then identified (second-level assessment). A nursing diagnosis follows, goals are set, and interventions are selected. Goals are mutually agreed on, and a goal-setting hierarchy is proposed. Survival is a priority goal, followed by goals that promote growth, ensure continuation of the species or society, and promote attainment of full potential. Factors precipitating ineffective behavior are changed, and coping behavior (i.e., adaptation level) is broadened. The person's level of coping is continuously revised. Evaluation of interventions requires returning to the first steps in the nursing process (i.e., noting behaviors manifested by the adaptive system or person).

J. G. PATERSON AND L. T. ZDERAD

Humanistic nursing, 1976

The person is a unique being, extant in all nursing situations, who innately struggles—to know. Humanistic nursing is an existential experience of being and doing so that nurturance with another occurs. Fundamentally, nursing is a response to human need that can be described to build a humanistic nursing science.

Humanistic nursing requires that the participants be aware of their uniqueness, as well as their commonality with others. Authenticity is required—an in-touchness with self that comes in part with experiencing. Humanistic nursing also presupposes responsible choices. The ability of an individual to make choices based on authentic awareness and knowledge of such choices is a concern of humanistic nursing and cultivates moreness. Also, a commitment to the value of humanistic nursing must be present.

A nurse with the foregoing attitudes and qualities can offer genuine presence to another. Humanistic nursing concerns the basic nursing act: the response of one human in need to another. At this level nursing is related to the health-illness quality of the human condition: nurturance toward more being.

M. M. LEININGER

Transcultural nursing: concepts, theories, and practices, 1978
Caring: a central focus of nursing and health care services, 1980
The phenomenon of caring: importance, research questions and theoretical considerations, 1981
Leininger's theory of nursing: cultural care diversity and universality, 1988

Caring is postulated as the central and unifying domain for nursing knowledge and practices. Diverse factors influence patterns of care and health or well-being in different cultures. Caring includes assistive, supportive, and facilitative acts for another individual or a group with evident or anticipated needs. Caring serves to ameliorate or to improve human conditions through behaviors, techniques, processes, and patterns. Professional nursing care embodies scientific and humanistic modes of helping or enabling receipt of personalized service to maintain a healthy condition for life or death.

Caring emphasizes healthful, enabling activities of individuals and groups that are based on culturally defined ascribed or sanctioned helping modes. Caring behaviors include comfort, compassion, concern, coping behavior, empathy, enabling, facilitating, interest, involvement, health-consultative acts, health-instruction acts, health-maintenance acts, helping behaviors, love, nurturance, presence, protective behaviors, restorative behaviors, sharing, stimulating behaviors, stress alleviation, succorance, support, surveillance, tenderness, touching, and trust (1981, p. 13). Culture determines personal life or worldviews that are mediated through language. Contextual factors such as technology, religion, philosophic beliefs, social and kinship lines and patterns, values and lifeways, political and legal factors, economic factors, and educational factors all influence care patterns. Likewise, these factors affect care patterns and the health of individuals and families, as well as groups. Diverse health systems mediate the expression of health. Nursing is one health system that overlaps with folk systems and professional health care systems.

Human caring is a universal phenomenon, and every nursing situation has transcultural nursing care elements. Caring is essential to human development, growth, and survival, and caring behaviors vary transculturally in priorities, expression, and needs satisfaction. Caring plays a more important role in recovery than cure but receives less reward. If effective, caring reflects professional concern, compassion, stress alleviation, nurturance, comfort, and protection. Nursing should provide care consistent with its emergent science and knowledge, with caring as a central focus. Caring and culture are inextricably linked, and nursing care should be culturally congruent and aimed at preserving, maintaining, accommodating, negotiating, repatterning, and restructuring care patterns.

J. WATSON

Nursing: the philosophy and science of caring, 1979
Nursing: human science and human care, 1985
New dimensions of human caring theory, 1988
Watson's philosophy and theory of human caring in nursing, 1989

Assumptions underlying human care values in nursing are (1) care and love comprise the primal and universal psychic energy and (2) care and love are requisite for our survival and the nourishment of humanity. Caring for and loving self is requisite to caring for others. Curing is not the end to be sought but is a means to care. Nursing's ability to sustain its caring ideology and translate it into practice will determine its contribution to society. Nursing has traditionally held a caring stance in relation to patients with health and illness concerns, and caring is the unifying focus for practice in nursing. Caring has received little emphasis in the health care system, and the caring values of nursing are critical to sustaining care ideals in practice. Preservation of human care is a significant issue, human care can be practiced only interpersonally, and nursing's social, moral, and scientific contributions lie in its commitment to human care ideals. The foregoing assumptions provide a rationale for developing nursing as a human science.

Humans are capable of transcending time and space, and each possesses a spirit, soul, or essence that enables self-awareness, higher degrees of consciousness, and a power to transcend the usual self. Human life is a continuous (with time and space) being in the world. Caring, an intersubjective human process, is the moral ideal of nursing. Human care processes have an energy field and involve engagement of mind-body-soul with another in a lived moment. Illness, not necessarily disease, is a state of subjective turmoil in which self as "I" is separated from self as "me." Conversely, health is a harmony within mind-body-soul in which the "I" and "me" are aligned. A healthy person is open to increased diversity. The goal of nursing is to help people increase harmony within mind-body-soul, which leads to self-knowledge, self-reverence, self-healing, and self-care.

Theoretic premises identified include the following: At nursing's highest level, the nurse makes contact with the person's emotional and subjective world as the route to inner self; mind and soul are not confined in time and space and to the physical universe; a nurse can access inner self through the mind-body-soul, provided the physical body is not perceived separate from the higher sense of self. The *geist* (spirit or inner self) exists in and for itself and relates to the human ability to be free; love and caring are universal givens; illness may be hidden from the "eyes" and requires finding meaning in inner experiences. Finally the totality of experiences at the moment constitute a phenomenal field or the individual's frame of reference.

Humans strive to satisfy needs experienced in the perceived phenomenal field, including being cared for, loved, and valued and experiencing positive regard, acceptance, and understanding. People also strive to achieve union, transcend individual life, and find harmony with life. All needs are subservient to a basic striving toward actualizing spiritual self and establishing harmony within mind-body-soul. Harmony is consistent with a sense of congruence between "I" and "me," between self as perceived and self as experienced, and between subjective reality (phenomenal field) and external reality (world as is).

Caring occasions involve action and choice by nurse and individual. If the caring occasion is transpersonal, the limits of openness and human capacities are expanded. Transpersonal caring relationships depend on (1) moral commitments to enhance human dignity to allow people to determine their own meaning, (2) the nurse's affirmation of the subjective significance of the person, (3) the nurse's ability to detect feelings of another's inner condition and feel a union with another, and (4) the nurse's history of living and experiencing feelings and human conditions and imagining others' feelings (that is, personal growth, maturation, and development of the nurse's self).

Nursing interventions related to human care are referred to as *carative* factors and include nurturing, forming, cultivating, and using (1) a humanistic-altruistic system of values; (2) faith-hope, (3) sensitivity to self and others; (4) helping-trusting human care relationship; (5) expressed positive and negative feelings; (6) a creative problem-solving caring process; (7) transpersonal teaching-learning; (8) supportive, protective, and/or corrective mental, physical, societal, and spiritual environment; (9) human needs assistance; and (10) existential-phenomenologic spiritual forces. Carative factors are actualized in the human care process.

M. A. NEWMAN

Theory development in nursing, 1979
Newman's health theory, 1983
Health as expanding consciousness, 1986

Individuals are subsumed by a greater whole and are part of multiple system levels in space. Explicit assumptions are made in relation to health, pathology, and patterns. Health can encompass pathology and disease; therefore, disease and health are not continuous variables or opposites. Pathology is manifested according to a pre-existing unitary pattern; thus disease gives clues to the pattern of a person's life, and pattern is reflected in energy exchange within humans and between humans and the environment. Personal patterns manifesting as disease are part of larger patterns, which are not altered when the disease is eliminated. Disease as a pattern manifestation may be considered health. The existence of disease may evoke tension, an important evolutionary ingredient. Disease is not advocated as a desirable state, but the significance of attending to the meaning of the disease is highlighted. Health is an expansion of consciousness, and pattern-manifesting disease expands consciousness.

Consciousness, the informational capacity of the system, is reflected in both the quality and quantity of responses to stimuli. Health involves developing awareness of self and environment, coupled with increased ability to perceive and respond to alternatives. Movement is a central concept, a property of life. The concepts of consciousness, time, movement, and space are interrelated in that movement reflects consciousness and is an identifiable and specific individual characteristic. Time is an index of consciousness and a function of movement. Movement is the means by which time and space become reality, and space and time have a complimentary relationship. Without movement, time and space are not real, and there is no change at any system level. Movement reflects the organization of consciousness and therefore reflects health. The implied goal is consciousness expansion and therefore health and life. Health is not a state but an experienced process.

D. E. JOHNSON

The behavioral system model for nursing, 1980

The individual patient is a behavioral system composed of subsystems. As a behavioral system, the patient's subsystems strive to maintain balance by making adjustments to factors impinging on them. Humans seek experiences that may disturb balance and require behavior modifications to reestablish balance. Behavioral systems are essential and reflect adaptations that are successful. The behavioral system is composed of behaviors that form an integrated unit. Behavioral systems maintain their own integrity, link individuals with environment, and are self-perpetuating if environmental conditions remain orderly and predictable. The multiple tasks of behavioral systems require continual system changes, including subsystem evolution. Subsystems also must be protected, nurtured, and stimulated.

Behavioral system subsystems are formed from responses or response tendencies that share a common goal and are modified by maturation and experience. Each subsystem of the overall behavioral system has a specialized task or function that can be described on the basis of that structure and function. There are four structural elements in each subsystem: (1) drive-stimulated or goal sought, (2) set or predisposition to act in a given way, (3) choices, or scope of action alternatives, and (4) behavior. Only the last structural element is observable. Seven subsystems are identified: (1) attachment or affiliative, (2) dependency, (3) ingestive, (4) eliminative, (5) sexual, (6) aggressive, and (7) achievement. The attachment subsystem responses provide security, and dependency provides for nurturance responses. The ingestive and eliminative subsystems relate to eating and excretion of waste. The sexual subsystem relates to the dual responses of procreation and sexual fulfillment. The aggressive subsystem functions to preserve the person, and the achievement system functions so that mastery of self and the environment is fostered.

Nursing problems are manifested when subsystems cannot maintain a dynamic stability or when the subsystem has not achieved an optimum level of function. Anticipated problems in subsystems can be prevented, and manifested problems can be solved. The nurse acts to impose a regulatory mechanism, change structural units, and fulfill functional requirements of subsystems. The nursing act seeks to "preserve the organization and integration of the patient's behavior at an optimal level under those conditions in which the behavior constitutes a threat to physical or social health, or in which illness is found" (p. 214).

R. R. PARSE

Man-living-health: a theory of nursing, 1981, 1989
Nursing science: major paradigms, theories and critiques, 1987

The person is unitary—that is, an indivisible being who interrelates with the environment while cocreating health. Theoretic assumptions synthesize the concepts of energy field, openness, pattern and organization, four dimensionality, helicy, integrality, coconstitution, coexistence, and situated freedom with tenets of human subjectivity and intentionality. Assumptions (nine in the 1981 book were reduced to three in the 1987 article) state that man is a recognizable pattern who evolves simultaneously with environment. Man-environment relationships are such that a continuity of what was and what will be unfolds in the now. Man chooses the meaning given to cocreated situations and is responsible for choices made. Unitary man is recognized by individual patterns of relating, which are cocreated in man-environment interchange. There is mutual man-environment interrelatedness as man chooses to move toward irreversible possibilities. Man experiences in multiple dimensions simultaneously and relatively. The negentropic interchange of man-environment both enables and limits becoming.

Health is an open process of becoming, an incarnation of man's choosings. As man and environment connect and separate, health is cocreated. Thus health is a synthesis of values cocreated in open interchange with environment. Health is a continuous process of transcending with the possibles— that is, reaching beyond the actual. Health is an emergent: a negentropic unfolding. The theory of man-living-health emerges from the stated assumptions, and three principles are notable: (1) structuring meaning multidimensionally is cocreating reality through the languaging of valuing and imaging, (2) cocreating rhythmic patterns of relating is living the paradoxical unity of revealing-concealing and enabling-limiting while connecting-separating, and (3) cotranscending with the possibles is powering unique ways or originating in the process of transforming (1987, p. 163).

Principle 1 asserts that reality is continually cocreated by assigning meaning to all-at-once experiences occurring multidimensionally. Imaging, valuing, and languaging serve to structure meaning multidimensionally. Principle 2 asserts that there is an unfolding cadence of coconstituting ways of being. Ways of being are recognized in the man-environment interchange and are lived rhythmically. Rhythms of revealing-concealing, enabling-limiting, and connecting-separating are integral in the principles. The final principle asserts that concepts of cotranscending with the possibles—powering, originating, and transforming—are man's ways of aspiring toward the "not-yet." Three theoretic structures are posited: (1) powering is a way of revealing and concealing imaging, (2) originating is a manifestation of enabling and limiting valuing, and (3) transforming unfolds in the languaging of connecting and separating (1981, p. 68).

P. BENNER AND J. WRUBEL

The primacy of caring, 1989

Caring is primary because it determines and constitutes what matters to people. Subsequently caring creates possibilities for coping (p. 3), enables possibilities for connecting with, and concern for, others (p. 4), and allows giving and receiving help (p. 4). Caring determines what is stressful to people and how they will cope.

Drawing on Heideggerian phenomenology, Benner and Wrubel posit a phenomenologic view of the person central to this view of caring. The person is a self-interpreting being who is defined by the process of living and being in the world. Through the process of living, people come to possess a nonreflective view of the self and can immediately grasp the meaning of a situation; that is, people understand the meaning of a context without conscious, deliberative reflection. This immediate grasping of situational meaning—self-interpretation—is possible because of the human characteristics of (1) embodied intelligence, (2) acquisition of background meaning, and (3) concern.

Embodied intelligence is the capacity of being in a situation in meaningful ways and effortlessly understanding it in relation to self. Background meanings are the cultural traditions "given" to a person from birth. These two features account for how people are in the world. Concern, the third characteristic of self-interpreting beings, accounts for why people are involved in the world in certain ways. These three characteristics are central to involvement with the world in ways that ensure people will grasp the meaning of situations in relation to the situation's meaning for them. Both nurse and client are self-interpreting beings. This view of the person as self-interpreting is central to understanding how caring and concern in nursing relate to understanding and facilitating stress-coping situations in patients.

People have both freedoms and constraints that result from the assumption that people are self-interpreting (i.e., their being is contextual or situational, and they interpret contexts in relation to self). In this view ordinary life experiences both create and determine stress and coping patterns of people. When illness and disease inevitably occur in the course of living, life contexts change and situational meanings alter. Old self-understandings do not work, a qualitatively different form of stress occurs, and the need for new patterns of coping emerges. New coping possibilities do exist in current situations, but these are understood in the context of old habits, skills, practices, and expectations (p. 23). These new possibilities and freedoms within the present contexts and situations (like the old possibilities and freedoms that no longer work) are not readily understood by the person.

Nursing is a process of helping people cope with the stress of illness, not by following sets of prescribed rules but by contextually dependent caring and concern. Understanding the illness experience of the patient is central to concern and caring. Illness is a central focus of nursing. Illness is not reducible to disease (cellular pathology), but it connotes human loss experiences and dysfunction precipitated by human loss. Because nursing concerns itself with the relationship between the disease process and the illness experience of self-interpreting beings, a concept of mind-body dualism is not possible.

Caring in the context of nursing depends on discerning problems, recognizing solutions, and helping patients implement, and live, a solution. Thus nursing is a moral act that goes beyond mere application of scientific knowledge. Understanding the illness experience of the person is central to helping an individual come to live meaningful coping processes and return to health. Being present for patients and expert interpretive skills facilitate concern as a vehicle for caring. Caring concern is central to human (nurse and patient) understanding of the situation of illness. Concern allows both nurse and patient to be in touch with the patient's lived experience. Emotions are a particular focus for concern because they are essential to patient and nurse understanding of the context of the patient, they provide clues to what is important in the situation, and they are linked to past experiences that need to be focused on and reinterpreted in the context of the present. This reinterpretation of past experiences and of old patterns of coping with life's inevitable stresses creates new contexts, and the situated freedoms and possibilities inherent in the present are more fully illuminated. New coping options result.

Because human beings can inhabit a common world with common meanings, common stress and coping patterns will exist. Phenomenologically grounded scientific study of stress and coping would reveal those common themes, meanings, and personal concerns as a basis for understanding caring practices in nursing.

Reference List

Abdellah FG, et al: *Patient-centered approaches to nursing,* New York, 1960, Macmillan.

Benner P, Wrubel J: *The primacy of caring,* Menlo Park, Calif, 1989, Addison-Wesley.

Hall LE: Another view of nursing care and quality. In Straub KM, Parker KS, editors: *Continuity in patient care: the role of nursing,* Washington, DC, 1966, Catholic University Press.

Henderson V: *The nature of nursing,* New York, 1966, Macmillan.

Johnson DE: The behavioral system model for nursing. In Riehl JP, Roy C, editors: *Conceptual models for nursing practice,* ed 2, New York, 1980, Appleton-Century-Crofts.

King IM: *Toward a theory for nursing: general concepts of human behavior,* New York, 1971, John Wiley & Sons.

King IM: *A theory for nursing: systems, concepts, process,* New York, 1981, John Wiley & Sons.

King IM: King's general systems framework and theory. In Riehl-Sisca J, editor: *Conceptual models for nursing practice,* ed 3, Norwalk, Conn, 1989, Appleton & Lange.

Leininger MM: *Transcultural nursing: concepts, theories, and practices,* New York, 1978, John Wiley & Sons.

Leininger MM: Caring: a central focus of nursing and health care services, *Nurs Health Care* 1:135, 1980.

Leininger MM: The phenomenon of caring: importance, research questions and theoretical considerations. In *Caring: an essential human need* (proceedings of the three national caring conferences), Thorofare, NJ, 1981, Charles B Slack.

Leininger MM: Leininger's theory of nursing: cultural care diversity and universality, *Nurs Sci Q* 1:152, 1988.

Levine ME: The four conservation principles of nursing, *Nurs Forum* 6:45, 1967.

Levine ME: *Introduction to clinical nursing,* ed 2, Philadelphia, 1973, FA Davis.

Levine ME: The conservation principles: twenty years later. In Riehl-Sisca J, editor: *Conceptual models for nursing practice,* ed 3, Norwalk, Conn, 1989, Appleton & Lange.

Neuman B: The Betty Neuman health care systems model: a total person approach to patient problems. In Riehl JP and Roy C, editors: *Conceptual models for nursing practice,* ed 2, New York, 1980, Appleton-Century-Crofts.

Neuman B: *The Neuman systems model,* Norwalk, Conn, 1982, Appleton-Century-Crofts.

Neuman B: *The Neuman systems model,* ed 2, Norwalk, Conn, 1989, Appleton & Lange.

Newman MA: *Theory development in nursing,* Philadelphia, 1979, FA Davis.

Newman MA: Newman's health theory. In Clements IW, Roberts FB, editors: *Family health: a theoretical approach to nursing care,* New York, 1983, John Wiley & Sons.

Newman MA: *Health as expanding consciousness,* St Louis, 1986, Mosby–Year Book.

Orem DE: *Nursing: concepts of practice,* New York, 1971, McGraw-Hill.

Orem DE: *Nursing: concepts of practice,* ed 2, New York, 1980, McGraw-Hill.

Orem DE: *Nursing: concepts of practice,* ed 3, New York, 1985, McGraw-Hill.

Orem DE: *Nursing: concepts of practice,* ed 4, St Louis, 1991, Mosby–Year Book.

Orlando IJ: *The dynamic nurse-patient relationship: function, process, and principles,* New York, 1961, GP Putman's Sons (republished in 1990 by the National League for Nursing).

Orlando IJ: *The discipline and teaching of nursing process: an evaluation study,* New York, 1972, GP Putnam's Sons.

Parse RR: *Man-living-health: a theory of nursing,* New York, 1981, John Wiley & Sons.

Parse RR: *Nursing science: major paradigms, theories and critiques,* Philadelphia, 1987, WB Saunders.

Parse RR: Man-living-health: a theory of nursing. In Riehl-Sisca J, editor: *Conceptual models for nursing practice,* ed 3, Norwalk, Conn, 1989, Appleton & Lange.

Paterson JG, Zderad LT: *Humanistic nursing,* New York, 1976, John Wiley & Sons (republished in 1987 by the National League for Nursing).

Peplau HE: *Interpersonal relations in nursing,* New York, 1952, GP Putnam's Sons.

Peplau HE: The art and science of nursing: similarities, differences, and relations, *Nurs Sci Q* 9:8, 1988.

Rogers ME: *An introduction to the theoretical basis of nursing,* Philadelphia, 1970, FA Davis.

Rogers ME: Nursing: a science of unitary man. In Riehl JP, Roy C, editors: *Conceptual models for nursing practice,* ed 2, New York, 1980, Appleton-Century-Crofts.

Rogers ME: Science of unitary human beings: a paradigm for nursing. In Clements IW, Roberts FB, editors: *Family health: a theoretical approach to nursing care,* New York, 1983, John Wiley & Sons.

Rogers ME: Nursing: a science of unitary human beings. In Riehl-Sisca J, editor: *Conceptual models for nursing practice,* ed 3, Norwalk, Conn, 1989, Appleton & Lange.

Roy C: *Introduction to nursing: an adaptation model,* Englewood Cliffs, NJ, 1976, Prentice-Hall.

Roy C: The Roy adaptation model. In Riehl JP, Roy C, editors: *Conceptual models for nursing practice,* ed 2, New York, 1980, Appleton-Century-Crofts.

Roy C: *Introduction to nursing: an adaptation model,* ed 2, Norwalk, Conn, 1984, Appleton-Century-Crofts.

Roy C: The Roy adaptation model. In Riehl-Sisca J, editor: *Conceptual models for nursing practice,* ed 3, Norwalk, Conn, 1989, Appleton & Lange.

Roy C, Roberts S: *Theory construction in nursing: an adaptation model,* Englewood Cliffs, NJ, 1981, Prentice-Hall.

Travelbee J: *Interpersonal aspects of nursing,* Philadelphia, 1966, FA Davis.

Travelbee J: *Interpersonal aspects of nursing,* ed 2, Philadelphia, 1971, FA Davis.

Watson J: *Nursing: the philosophy and science of caring,* Boston, 1979, Little, Brown (republished in 1988 by the National League for Nursing).

Watson J: *Nursing: human science and human care,* Norwalk, Conn, 1985, Appleton-Century-Crofts.

Watson J: New dimensions of human caring theory, *Nurs Sci Q* 9:175, 1988.

Watson J: Watson's philosophy and theory of human caring in nursing. In Riehl-Sisca J, editor: *Conceptual models for nursing practice,* ed 3, Norwalk, Conn, 1989, Appleton & Lange.

Wiedenbach E: *Clinical nursing: a helping art,* New York, 1964, Springer.

Appendix B

Interpretive Summary: Selected Midrange Theories

The summaries provided here provide examples of midrange theories in nursing. They are not complete descriptions or critical reflections of the theorists' works, but rather they are interpretive descriptions of the essential features of the emerging theories. A notation of the definitive theoretic writing precedes the summary.

E. T. PATTERSON AND E. S. HALE

A Theory of Menstrual Care Activities of Daily Living
**Making sure: integrating menstrual care practices
into activities of daily living, 1985**

This is derived from a grounded theory study to inductively develop a substantive theory about integrating menstrual care practices into daily activities. Making sure, the core concept of the theory, is defined as the process that enables menstruating women to continue their daily activities, knowing that their practices of menstrual care are effective and that the menstrual care demand can be met efficiently and effectively. Accidents are errors in making sure. Day of flow is a condition affecting making sure. Backup mechanisms are the strategies used to enhance making sure. Public and private are the contexts affecting making sure. Attending, calculating, and juggling are the subprocesses of making sure. Attending is the process of assessing the current menstrual demand. Calculating is a cognitive process of placing the menstrual care demand within the broader system of daily care demands that results in a decision about what to do with respect to menstrual self-care. Juggling is the process of assuring that time, space, and supplies coincide to meet menstrual self-care demands. The concepts of the theory are analogous to the concepts of Orem's general theory of self-care (1980).

Making sure is composed of the three subprocesses of attending, calculating, and juggling. The three subprocesses occur in stages that are sequential phases of the core process of making sure; they are analogous to Orem's estimative, transitional, and productive operation of self-care (1980). Making sure occurs in the context of accidents, day of flow, backup mechanisms, and public and private contexts. The context of the theory is that surrounding menstruating women and consists of cultural, social, and personal values regarding menstruation.

The theory was inductively generated with a grounded theory methodology. Interviews were conducted with 25 women who volunteered or were invited to participate because of theoretically relevant variables. In addition to the interviews, informal anecdotes and serendipitous sampling were used—stories volunteered by friends and colleagues or overheard conversations in public restrooms. The process of data analysis involved coding, memoing, and sorting; ongoing comparison of incidents and codes was done to collapse categories into higher-level categories.

The purpose for developing this theory was to provide insight into nursing care that can enhance a woman's self-care ability, particularly in the early experience with menstruation. The theory has implications for education related to self-care activities, particularly with anticipating menarche and in preventing toxic shock syndrome. Further development of the theory is advocated by systematically applying the theory in practice. The authors also note that the theory may have applicability in other circumstances involving involuntary eliminative processes, such as occurs with an ostomy, urinary incontinence, or lactation.

L. R. PHILLIPS AND V. F. REMPUSHESKI

A Theory of Quality of Family Caregiving
Caring for the frail elderly at home: toward a theoretical explanation of the dynamics of poor quality family caregiving, 1986

This is a grounded-theory approach to theory development to inductively describe dynamics of good-quality and poor-quality family caregiving, explain the relationships among contextual and perceptual variables in caring for the elderly at home, and identify points at which interventions by nurses could be effective. Five major constructs were identified. *Personal identity* of the elder was defined as a mental image that the caregiver has of the elder being cared for. *Image of caregiving* was defined as the degree to which the caregiver's personal imperatives, standards, and values are realized by the caregiving situation. Caregiver's *role beliefs* were defined as the standards and values the caregiver held regarding the performance of the caregiver role; they include the caregiver's and the elder's expectations for role responsibilities. Caregiver *behavioral strategies* were defined as the behavior the caregiver customarily uses in responding to the elder. *Perception* is defined as the caregiver's interpretation of the elder's response.

The five major concepts of the theory were structured as stages consistent with the framework of symbolic interactionism. Stage 1, defining the process, consists of the personal identity of the elder and image of the caregiving. Stage 2, cognitive processes, consists of the caregiver's role beliefs. Stage 3, expressive processes, consists of the caregiver's behavioral strategies. Stage 4, evaluation processes, consists of perception.

The stage 1 construct of personal identity of the elder involves the associated concept of reconciliation of past with present, which in turn involves six distinct processes, each of which involves three separate steps of deriving a past image, deriving a present image, and reconciling past and present by using comparison. The reconciled image can be normalized or anormalized. Anormalized images can be either deified (viewing the elder as more adequate than is real) or stigmatized (viewing the elder as less adequate than is real).

The stage 1 construct of image of the caregiving involves the associated concept of reconciliation of proscriptions with the perceived reality of caregiving, or the degree to which the caregiver's observations and perceptions of the situation diverge from the caregiver's beliefs about propriety. Several interrelated categories of proscriptions are derived in the theory development process.

The stage 1 constructs have a direct influence on the stage 2 construct of the caregiver's role beliefs, which has two associated concepts: role responsibilities of the caregiver and role responsibilities of the elder. The nature of the influence between the two stages is a major factor in determining the quality of caregiving.

The stage 3 construct, the caregiver's behavioral strategies, involves the concept of the caregiver's management strategies or the methods used to control the elder's behavior and to resolve conflicts with the elder. Three types of management strategies were identified: positive, negative, and neutral.

The stage 4 construct of perception involves the concept of perception of the elder's response, or the caregiver's interpretation of the elder's role support and role enactment. This process, over time, can positively or negatively modify stage 1.

Details of the structure and context of the theory are presented in diagrams and clarified by definitions and examples from the data.

The theory was inductively generated with a grounded-theory methodology. In-depth interviews were conducted with 39 caregivers in two geographic locations who responded to one of two newspaper advertisements. One advertisement solicited caregivers who had a good relationship with an elder for whom they cared, and the other solicited caregivers who had an abusive or neglectful relationship with the elder. Approximately 2000 large data bits comprised the beginning working sample, which was derived from the interviews. The data were subjected to constant comparative analysis, consisting of open and selective coding.

The authors state that therapeutic and cost-effective care for elders depends on the nurse's understanding of the dynamics of family caregiving and on knowing how to intervene to meet the needs of both the elder and the family members who are providing care. The hypotheses generated in this study provide the basis for further testing of the theory in practice, which can lead to the ability to predict caregivers who are at high risk for providing less than optimal care and to identify those points at which interventions by nurses will be most effective in high-risk caregiving situations.

M. A. WEWERS AND E. R. LENZ

A Theory of Relapse among Ex-Smokers
**Relapse among ex-smokers: an example
of theory derivation, 1987**

This is a theory of relapse among ex-smokers derived from a theory of recovery from alcohol abuse; empiric testing of the derived theory with a prospective one-group-only design. Relapse is a central focus of the theory. The meaning of relapse among ex-smokers evolved from examining studies of the role of a specific factor in the relapse process and of alcohol relapse. Six factors that influence relapse were identified: sociodemographic and pretreatment smoking characteristics, nature of treatment received, and three posttreatment characteristics (stressors, coping responses, and family environment).

Relapse, the central concept of the theory, was postulated to be a function of three characteristics: patient-related characteristics, treatment-related characteristics, and posttreatment characteristics. Patient-related characteristics are the subfactors of sociodemographic factors and pretreatment symptoms. There were no subfactors for treatment-related characteristics. Subfactors under the concept of posttreatment characteristics were stressors, coping responses, and family environment.

Patient-related characteristics of sociodemographic factors, pretreatment symptoms, and the posttreatment characteristics of stressors, coping responses, and family environment were postulated to have a major explanatory role in the theory. Because of empiric evidence that countered any differential effect of various treatment techniques, treatment-related characteristics were assigned a minor explanatory role.

The context of ex-smokers was postulated to differ from the derived context of alcohol recovery in terms of the nature of stressful life events and physiologic factors arising from within the individual.

A study was conducted to examine the relationships between smoking relapse and five of the six major components of the theory with a one-group-only prospective design with 150 adults attending a smoking-cessation clinic. Variables that operationalized the theory factors were measured prior to beginning the treatment and then 3 months later. The results of the study suggested that the role of posttreatment characteristics, stressors (particularly craving), and type of coping response may be useful in designing effective treatments to prevent relapse.

The purpose underlying the development of this theory was to assist nurses in designing effective treatments to help ex-smokers maintain long-term abstinence and prevent relapse. The results of this empiric test of the derived theory suggested two major areas of focus for application of the theory. First, symptoms of craving should be considered a high-risk predictor of relapse. Second, a focus on problem-versus emotion-focused coping responses may improve success rates.

M. H. MISHEL

A Theory of Uncertainty
Reconceptualization of the uncertainty in illness theory, 1990

This is a reconceptualization of uncertainty theory (Mishel, 1988) to include experiences of living with continual uncertainty processes. Reconceptualization is based on an examination of theory and prior empiric evidence, with particular attention to the outcome portion of the theory. The original version of the uncertainty theory includes the major concept of uncertainty, which is the inability to determine the meaning of illness because cues necessary to assigning value are insufficient. Therefore, outcome of illness events cannot be known.

Two subconcepts that identify processes for appraisal of illness events precipitating uncertainty are inference and illusion. *Inference* is the construction of meaning by reference to exemplary former situations. *Illusion* refers to construction of a generally positive belief system.

Two subconcepts defining outcomes of appraisal processes are identified: danger and opportunity. For the appraisal process outcome of danger, two coping strategies are identified: mobilizing and affect-control strategies. For the appraisal process outcome of opportunity, the coping strategy of buffering is identified.

Adaptation, in the original version of the model, is identified as the outcome of all coping strategies, whether in response to uncertainty appraisal as danger or opportunity. Adaptation is a positive value and connotes stability and the return to equilibrium.

In the reformulated version of uncertainty theory, the concept of continual self-organization to increasing levels of complexity replaces adaptation as the outcome of uncertainty appraisal in situations of continuing and chronic uncertainty.

A structure of the outcome portion of an earlier version of the uncertainty theory (Mishel, 1988) is provided. A narrative also explains and adds structure to the visual of the earlier version, as well as the reformulated version of the theory. The structure is a time-ordered linear framework that begins with the situation of uncertainty in illness. Uncertainty is appraised by two processes: inference or illusion. The theory is structured so that both processes are influenced by (1) the patient, (2) the patient's social resources, and (3) health care providers. Inference, or comparison of present situations with earlier situations, can result in appraisal of uncertainty as either danger or opportunity. Illusion, or the construction of a belief system that is positive, usually results in a view of uncertainty as opportunity. Whether appraised as danger or as opportunity, coping with uncertainty follows its appraisal. If appraised as danger, coping strategies seek to decrease uncertainty. If appraised as opportunity, coping maintains uncertainty. Two strategies to decrease uncertainty are structured: mobilizing or affect-control strategies. Strategies to maintain uncertainty are structured to include buffering strategies.

In the earlier version of the theory, which was developed in the context of acute illness with a generally downward course, adaptation was the outcome of coping. Adaptation was assumed to be a positive state in which uncertainty was successfully manipulated in the desired direction. Adaptation constituted the end point of the theory.

The original theory was structured to include cultural biases inherent in the Western worldview. Assumptions reflecting this bias were identified to include (1) a temporal invariability in the appraisal of uncertainty, (2) uncertainty is generally aversive, and (3) uncertainty is a stable state rather than a process. The author states that this bias is reflected in prior research findings and limits advancing the theory. The reformulation of the theory challenges these assumptions and utilizes theory derivation as described by Walker and Avant (1989).

The theory is reformulated for the context of long-term chronic uncertainty situations. In long-term illness situations the early acute disruptions that create uncertainty and a high level of instability provide the foundation for evolving a new sense of order within the human system. Chaos theory is the perspective borrowed for reformulation of the outcome portion of the uncertainty theory. New levels of self-organization become the end point or the continuing process in response to the uncertainty of chronic illness.

The reformulation also discards the concept of illusion as a way to appraise uncertainty and the possibility of appraising uncertainty as negative or as danger. Rather, the theory is structured so that uncertainty as opportunity is the view maintained by the environmental forces of support resources and health care providers. Four factors are identified that block re-evaluation of uncertainty and continual self-organization to higher levels of complexity. These blocks occur when (1) patients' supportive resources do not promote a probabilistic view of life, (2) the patient caretakes others, (3) the patient is isolated from social interactional contexts, and (4) providers focus on certainty and definite illness outcomes. Blocks to the continual reintegration of uncertainty to new levels of self-organization can result in posttraumatic stress syndrome.

The reconceptualization of uncertainty theory is grounded in assumptions inherent in chaos theory that characterize far-from-equilibrium systems. The theory undergoing reconceptualization was the result of approximately 10 years of ongoing empiric research and theory formulation in a variety of health and illness contexts. The author suggests the need for empiric research for the newly reformulated theory. Also, practical use of the theory is suggested to promote a view of the uncertainty of life and the need to create unpredictable contingencies from seemingly unrelated situations.

The author does not specifically address research strategies for deliberative application aside from the suggested need for empiric research. Deliberative application might be accomplished through clinical application of the theory, with subsequent theory reformulation based on careful analysis of the experiences of clinicians.

A. A. QUINN

A Theory of Perimenopausal Process
A theoretical model of the perimenopausal process, 1991

This is a qualitative study to generate theory related to women's experience of perimenopausal processes. A core variable and four subprocesses emerged from data analysis. The core variable of integrating a changing me was the central concept. Four subprocesses were identified: (1) tuning in to me (my body and moods represented awareness of physical and emotional changes), (2) facing a paradox of feelings included negative and positive feelings about the menopausal experience, (3) contrasting impressions included processes of resolving conflicting information about the menopause, and (4) making adjustments referred to changes and alterations made in response to life changes. Subprocesses were further defined by narrative discussion that included examples and delineation of additional subprocesses.

A theoretic structure of a pinwheel was provided. The core variable (integrating a changing me) was located at the center. The four subprocesses were integrated and linked with the core variable. The subprocesses were not depicted as sequential or linear. The subprocesses were further structured as follows: Tuning in to me included processes of changing control and uncertainty in relation to qualitative and quantitative changes surrounding the menstrual cycle, hot flashes, breast tenderness, weight fluctuation, skin character, energy levels, and moods. Facing a paradox of feelings included both negative and positive feelings around getting older, reproduction, physical vulnerability, and the uncertainty of the future. Contrasting impressions were structured to include processing conflicting information about menopause acquired from stories, communication with others, exposure to media, and self-beliefs. Making adjustments included self-care practices to maintain health, coping strategies to handle stress, and caring activities. Making adjustment processes were further structured into changing diets, exercising, taking vitamins and calcium, creating time for self, making life accommodations, seeking solitude, promoting change, recognizing physical limits, putting lives in perspective, and regaining control. Further structure was provided throughout by use of examples and quotes from participants.

The theory was contextualized for the perimenopausal process as experienced by women. The structuring assumed (1) menopause was a natural process, (2) meaning attributed to the process was culturally based, (3) women's health is not synonymous with reproductive health, and (4) women's self-reports of their experience had validity.

The theory was generated with a grounded-theory methodology. Two main questions were asked: What is the process of menopause for perimenopausal women? What are the self-care practices used for? Perimenopause was defined as the cognitive, affective, and behavioral/physical responses of women aged 40 to 60. Self-care practices were defined as consistent with the self-care theory of Dorothea Orem (1980) to maintain life, health, and well-being.

Twelve women who were not on hormone therapy and who had varied backgrounds of marital status, education, and parity participated in the study. Women were interviewed and kept daily logs for 2 months. Field notes also contributed data. Theoretic sampling was used throughout data generation and analysis. Data were coded, categorized, and sorted by ethnographs to produce the core variable and related subprocesses. The truth value was established by confirming study findings with the women experiencing the perimenopausal process.

The author suggests use of the theory to understand the perimenopausal process and facilitate women's integration of the process. Providing a forum for women to express their concerns, share their stories, and receive information about the experience is cited as a clinical application of the theory. The use of the clinician's experience in applying the theory to subsequently expand and refine it could represent deliberative application processes, although this is not suggested by the author. The author does suggest further research in a variety of cultural and socioeconomic groups to broaden and expand the beginning theory.

P. G. REED

A Theory of Self-Transcendence
Toward a nursing theory of self-transcendence: deductive reformulation using developmental theories, 1991b

Using deductive reformulation as method for developing theory, the author reformulated life-span developmental theory from psychology, based on Rogers's general conceptual system of nursing. The definition of self-transcendence was based on reformulation that focused on areas of incongruence between life span development theory and Rogers's conceptual system for nursing. Self-transcendence was defined as expansion of self-boundaries multidimensionally—inwardly, outwardly, and temporally. Inward expansion involves introspective experience. Outward expansion involves reaching out to others. In temporal expansion past and future are integrated in the present. Self-transcendence is related conceptually to well-being, particularly in terms of mental health.

The structure and context of theory are expressed in two propositions that are set forth as central to the theory: (1) Self-transcendence is greater in persons facing end-of-own-life issues than in persons not confronted with such issues, and (2) self-transcendence is positively related to indicators of well-being in persons facing end-of-own-life issues.

The propositions of the theory were tested in five studies by Reed (1986a, 1986b, 1987, 1989, 1991a) that examined spiritual and psychosocial self-transcendence. The people who participated in these studies were either terminally ill adults or middle-old and eldest-old adults. The author developed a Spiritual Perspective Scale to measure multidimensional personal boundary expansion and a self-transcendence scale to measure psychosocial expressions of self-transcendence in later life. In addition to the quantitative analyses, qualitative data were analyzed by matrix analysis. The findings of all of the studies supported the initial propositions of the theory and provided a beginning empiric base for the theory.

The theory provides a rationale for nurses to attend to spiritual and psychosocial expressions of self-transcendence with clients who are experiencing end-of-own-life issues. The author notes that nursing therapies to help clients expand self-boundaries need to be tested in clinical practice. Potential approaches to nursing care that could be used in deliberative application include meditation, self-reflection, visualization, religious expression, peer counseling, journal keeping, and life-review processes.

K. M. SWANSON

A Theory of Caring in Perinatal Nursing
Empirical development of a middle-range theory of caring, 1991

This is an inductively developed theory of caring derived from three perinatal contexts. Caring is a central concept. Conceptual meaning was derived from empiric (phenomenologically based) study. The meaning of caring was expressed as five caring processes, each with four or five subprocesses. A discussion of each process further clarified meaning. An empirically based definition of caring was proposed. Conceptual meaning was validated by comparison with theoretic writings of Patricia Benner (1984), Nel Noddings (1984), and Jean Watson (1985).

Theory is structured in tabular form as five distinct but overlapping processes that define caring in the context of study. These five processes are (1) knowing, (2) being with, (3) doing for, (4) enabling, and (5) maintaining belief. Subdimensions that further define each process are listed. The narrative discussion and the empirically derived definition of caring provide further structure for the dimensions of caring.

The context of derivation was perinatal nursing. Three subcontexts from which the theory was structured were (1) women who recently miscarried, (2) caregivers in a newborn intensive care unit, and (3) young mothers at social risk.

The theory was generated by successive phenomenologically based studies within separate but related contexts. Women who miscarried were interviewed, and the five dimensions of caring emerged. Successive studies confirmed and refined the dimensions of caring that had emerged from the initial study. The second study utilized participant observation of care providers, attendance at ethics grand rounds, and interviews with various care providers, including nurses, physicians, fathers, mothers, an ethicist, a nursing administrator, and a social worker.

Deductive testing of the theory is in process. Women who have miscarried are receiving counseling grounded in the theory of caring. Outcomes related to healing and the meaning of the human experience of health and illness will be assessed.

The generation and testing operations that gave rise to the theory constituted deliberately applying theory because the initial study formed the basis for second and third deliberative attempts to modify and strengthen the theory.

Cross-validation of the theory was provided by comparison of the emerging theory with work of Nel Noddings (1984), Patricia Benner (1984), and Jean Watson (1985).

Deliberative application is proposed for other contexts of caring to determine the generalizability of the theory. Findings that suggest congruence with nonnursing theories of caring support generalizability to nonnursing contexts.

J. M. HITCHCOCK AND H. S. WILSON

A Theory of Personal Risking
Personal risking: lesbian self-disclosure of sexual orientation to professional health care providers, 1992

This is an inductively developed theory of sexual identity disclosure processes of lesbians seeking traditional health care. The basic social process of personal risking is a central concept. Conceptual meaning was derived from in-depth interviews and from the assignment of meaning with grounded-theory methodology. The meaning of personal risking is expressed through a series of complex conceptual networks of subconcepts representing processes and states related to personal risking.

Personal risking is conceptually divided into two phasic processes, which are both further defined by two subprocesses. Interactional stance is also an important concept and is defined by four subconcepts. Three additional concepts modify and determine the entire personal risking process: (1) personal attributes, (2) health care context, and (3) relevancy.

Conceptual meaning is provided by narrative description and examples from participants included in the report.

The concept of fear emerged as a basic social-psychologic problem that motivates the personal risking process.

The theoretic structure is derivable from the narrative. The basic social process of personal risking is a central concept. Personal risking is structured into two phases: (1) an anticipatory phase and (2) an interactional phase. The anticipatory phase is structured into two subprocesses: imagining scenarios and cognitive strategizing. Cognitive strategizing is substructured as formalizing and scouting out. Imagining scenarios is not further structured by subprocesses. Interactional stance is substructured into four concepts: (1) passive disclosure, (2) active disclosure, (3) passive nondisclosure, and (4) active nondisclosure. It also has two subprocesses: (a) scanning and (b) monitoring. Scanning occurs prior to contact with the provider. Monitoring occurs in the context of care provision.

Three additional concepts modify and determine the entire personal risking process: (1) personal attributes, (2) health care context, and (3) relevance. These concepts overlie the entire personal risking process. Personal attributes are structured to include the comfort level of the lesbian with sexual orientation, the relationship status of the lesbian, and the attitudes and beliefs about health care. Health care context includes provider characteristics (sexual orientation, gender, personal and professional attributes, the client's past experiences with providers), the health care environment, its location, and cues to its friendliness.

A linear structure for the major concepts is suggested in that the anticipatory phase is followed by the interactional phase. The concept of interactional stance is an outcome of the anticipatory phase, and interactional stance is implemented following the scanning process of the interactional phase. The interactional stance is continuously monitored during the implementation phase, with a feedback loop to interactional stance implied. The structure of the theory needs to consider stance modification (except if the stance of active disclosure has been implemented), depending on personal attributes, health care context, and relevance of disclosure.

The concept of fear emerged as a basic social-psychologic problem that helped focus the structuring of the theory; fear is shared by all participants and becomes a focus for the basic social process. Thus the resolution or management of fear becomes a focal point for theoretic organization in that the basic social process of personal risking can be organized to show how it relates to the management of fear.

The theory was contextualized in relation to traditional health care environment processes and providers as experienced by lesbian women of broad ranges of age, income level, and years of formal education. The contextual variable of relationship status was also operating in that relationship status was not controlled.

The theory was inductively generated with a grounded-theory methodology. One-time in-depth interviews of participants were the source of data. A three-step coding process was used in data analysis. Level 1 codes were substantive codes that described experiences in the participant's own words. Level 2 codes were applied to initial clusters of level 1 data. Level 3 codes were those applied to the core concepts of the theory.

This is implied in suggestions for further development, which could accrue through deliberative application of the theory or focus on the theory-development process: generation and testing of theoretic relationships. Deliberative application in different contexts—for example, geographic location and ethnicity of respondents—would further define the context and provide information on generalizability of the findings. The authors suggest a theory-verifying approach for exploring conditions of personal attributes, health care context, and relevance (particularly the effect each has on the personal risking process). Deliberative application also needs to focus on the reality of health care provider attitudes toward lesbian health issues and how they affect personal risking processes.

C. L. WIENER AND M. J. DODD

A Theory of Illness Trajectory
Coping amid uncertainty: an illness trajectory perspective, 1993

This is a secondary analysis of qualitative data for congruity with an extant theoretic framework of illness trajectory; a test of the validity of this theoretic framework with cancer patients by interrelating concepts of illness trajectory, coping, and uncertainty. Illness trajectory is a central concept and names the theoretic framework to be validated. The meaning of illness trajectory evolved from studies of chronically ill people that began in the 1960s and continued through the late 1980s. *Illness trajectory* is defined loosely as the path of an illness course and is further defined by three major subconcepts.

The course of the disease refers to an individual's life course of living with a chronic illness, which is additionally defined by three major concepts.

Other key concepts are coping and uncertainty. The meaning of coping, as a correlate of stress, is consistent with the usage in Patricia Benner's caring theory (1989). The dimensions of uncertainty evolved from extensive qualitative data analysis.

The illness trajectory theory is more specifically defined as work done over the total course of the disease. There are three subconcepts or dimensions of work done: (1) the physical unfolding of the disease, (2) the total organization of work done over the course of the disease, and (3) the reciprocal consequences for family, health care professionals, and patients. The framework is undergirded by an assumption that work occurs in a social context. Subsequent research with the illness trajectory framework identified three interrelated elements around the course of a disease as a life course: (1) conceptions of self and (2) evolution of self over time that (3) arise directly or indirectly from the body. The theoretic structure is consistent with the expectation that these three life course concepts work together to provide structure and continuity to living. The need for coping arises when illness, such as cancer, intrudes.

The theory developed from this base and reported in this research derived from the examination of the uncertainty data in relation to temporality, body, and identity—concepts directly related to the elements of subconcepts around the life course of disease. Three major concepts evolved: uncertain temporality, uncertain body, and uncertain identity. The dimensions of uncertain temporality include (1) loss of temporal predictability (duration, pace, frequency of recurrence), (2) sketching out and constriction of time, and (3) time as limitless. These dimensions were correlates of patient concern about the efficacy of treatment, recurrence of illness, unreliability of symptoms, and risk inherent in treatment. The dimensions of the uncertain body included: (1) body failure (activity performance, appearance, physiologic function) and (2) the body's response to treatment. These dimensions correlated with patient concerns with new bodily symptoms, with having the body's resistance in jeopardy, and with what was being done with the body. The uncertain identity arises through the body and the challenges to who the patient is.

These theoretic dimensions that evolved from interrelating uncertainty with one major facet of the illness trajectory (the life course of a disease) formed a basis for examining the second major concept of the illness (work done over this life course). This resulted in the structuring of four major concepts: illness-related work, everyday work, biographic work, and uncertainty-abatement work. Illness-related work included symptom management, following the management regimen, crisis prevention and management, and diagnostic-related work. Everyday work included housekeeping and repairing, occupational work, marital, child rearing, recreation, and daily living activities. Biographic work included gathering and dispensing information, expressing concern, caring, anger; and dividing tasks. Uncertainty-abatement work included pacing, becoming a professional patient, seeking reinforcing comparisons, engaging in reviews, setting goals, covering up, finding a safe place to let down, choosing a supportive network, and taking charge.

Uncertainty is both a response to and an outcome of work and life course processes within the illness trajectory. Coping is also a response to and outcome of uncertainty. Thus the concepts of coping, uncertainty, and illness trajectory are structurally interrelated to allow mutual, simultaneous interaction.

The theory derived from this research is contextualized for patients with an initial or ongoing cancer diagnosis who require chemotherapy and for their families.

Utilizing the borrowed theoretic framework of illness trajectory, uncertainty was examined in light of its three elements. Uncertainty data were part of a larger study of family coping and self-care during 6 months of a chemotherapy experience. The core variable of "tolerating the uncertainty that permeates the disease" emerged from qualitative data analysis. This research examined the work processes (that define the concept of illness trajectory) of coping in the face of uncertainty.

The uncertainty data examined were accrued from 100 interviews of a family member of a variety of patients with cancer. Each family member was interviewed 3 times during a 6-month period of chemotherapy, either initial or repeated. The authors acknowledge that the re-examination of existing data from the perspective of grounded-theory methodology departs from its original intent. The coding paradigm was adapted to retrospective data to elicit the dimensions of uncertainty and the management processes people use to deal with cancer and its consequences.

Deliberative application is suggested in relation to theoretic sampling under different cultural conditions or among patients with different chronic illnesses. Inherent in these suggestions is sampling with patients for whom uncertainty has varying significance.

That health care professionals use insights to provide care suggests the possibility for intervention studies to determine if nursing care deliberately structured to manage uncertainty and facilitate coping would have reciprocal positive effects on these experiences.

Reference List

Benner P: *From novice to expert: excellence and power in clinical nursing practice,* Menlo Park, Calif, 1984, Addison-Wesley.

Benner P, Wrubel J: *The primacy of caring,* Menlo Park, Calif, 1989, Addison-Wesley.

Hitchcock JM, Wilson HS: Personal risking: lesbian self-disclosure of sexual orientation to professional health care providers, *Nurs Res* 41:178, 1992.

Mishel MH: Uncertainty in illness, *Image* 20:225, 1988.

Mishel MH: Reconceptualization of the uncertainty in illness theory, *Image* 22:256, 1990.

Noddings N: *Caring: a feminine approach to ethics and moral education,* Berkeley, 1984, University of California Press.

Orem D: *Nursing: concepts of practice,* ed 2, New York, 1980, McGraw-Hill.

Patterson ET, Hale ES: Making sure: integrating menstrual care practices into activities of daily living, *Adv Nurs Sci* 7:18, 1985.

Phillips LR, Rempusheski VF: Caring for the frail elderly at home: toward a theoretical explanation of the dynamics of poor quality family caregiving, *Adv Nurs Sci* 8:62, 1986.

Quinn AA: A theoretical model of the perimenopausal process, *J Nurs Midwife* 36:25, 1991.

Reed PG: Developmental resources and expression in the elderly, *Nurs Res* 35:368, 1986a.

Reed PG: Religiousness among terminally ill and healthy adults, *Res Nurs Health* 9:35, 1986b.

Reed PG: Spirituality and well-being in terminally ill hospitalized adults, *Res Nurs Health* 10:335, 1987.

Reed PG: Mental health of older adults, *West J Nurs Res* 11:143, 1989.

Reed PG: Self-transcendence and mental health in oldest-old adults, *Nurs Res* 40:1, 1991a.

Reed PG: Toward a nursing theory of self-transcendence: deductive reformulation using developmental theories, *Adv Nurs Sci* 13:64, 1991b.

Swanson KM: Empirical development of a middle-range theory of caring, *Nurs Res* 40:161, 1991.

Walker LO, Avant KC: *Strategies for theory construction in nursing,* ed 2, Norwalk, Conn, 1989, Appleton-Century-Crofts.

Watson J: *Nursing: human science and human care,* Norwalk, Conn, 1985, Appleton-Century-Crofts.

Wewers MA, Lenz ER: Relapse among ex-smokers: an example of theory derivation, *Adv Nurs Sci* 9:44, 1987.

Wiener CL, Dodd MJ: Coping amid uncertainty: an illness trajectory perspective, *Scholar Inq Nurs Pract* 7:17, 1993.

Glossary

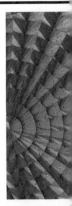

abstract concept Mental image derived largely from indirect evidence that is not easily presented by a specific empiric indicator.

accessibility Trait of theory useful for questioning and clarifying the degree to which concepts have indicators in observable reality and, subsequently, how attainable are the outcomes, goals, and purposes of the theory.

aesthetics Fundamental pattern of knowing in nursing related to the perception of deep meanings, calling forth inner creative resources that transform experience into what is not yet real, but possible. Expressed as knowledge through works of art and criticism and integrated in practice as transformative art-acts.

appreciation Process of focusing and reflecting on aesthetic knowledge as it is understood and valued by members of the discipline. Interacts with the process of inspiration to challenge and authenticate aesthetic knowledge.

assumption One of the structural components of theory that is taken for granted or thought to be true without systematically generated empiric evidence. Theoretic assumptions may be value statements or have potential for empiric testing but are assumed true within the theory because they are reasonable.

atomistic theory Theory that deals with a narrow scope of phenomena. The term often implies, in addition, an assumption that the whole may be understood from a study of the parts.

axiom Type of premise used in deductive logic, often one that is not tentative but relatively firm. Axioms as premises are used for deducing theorems, especially in mathematics.

centering Process that involves a deliberate focus on inner feelings, perception, and experience and involves contemplation and introspection to form deep inner personal meaning from life experiences. Interacts with the process of opening to create personal knowledge.

clarifying Process involving a deliberate focus on understanding the nature of ethical decisions and dilemmas and on bringing to full understanding those actions that are right and good. Interacts with the process of valuing to create ethical knowledge.

251

clarity Trait of theory useful for questioning and understanding the degree to which a theory is semantically and structurally lucid and consistent.

codes A form of knowledge expression within the ethics pattern. Codes are shorthand expressions of prescribed professional behaviors that are generally accepted as right and good. Codes primarily describe behaviors that represent the nurse's accountability to the client as expressed in rights, duties, and obligations.

components of theory Features of theory that are useful for describing theory and that form a template for critically reflecting theory. Components include purpose, concepts, definitions, relationships, structure, and assumptions.

concept Complex mental formulation of experience. Concepts are a major component of theory and convey the abstract ideas within the theory.

conceptual framework A logical grouping of related concepts or theories, usually created to draw together several different aspects that are relevant to a complex situation such as a practice setting or an educational program. Term used synonymously with theoretic framework. A knowledge form within the empirics pattern.

conclusions Relationship statements that are derived from premises in a deductive logic system. Conclusions are a type of proposition and may take the form of a theorem or hypothesis.

consistency Trait related to clarity. Consistency may be semantic or structural and refers to the general agreement, harmony, and compatibility of components within the theory.

construct Type of highly abstract and complex concept whose reality base can be only inferred. Constructs are formed from multiple less abstract or more empiric concepts.

creating conceptual meaning Theory development process of identifying, examining, and clarifying the mental images that comprise the elements, variables, or concepts within theory. Conveys the thoughts, feelings, and ideas that reflect the human experience of the concept.

criteria for concepts Essential features of a concept formed by examining conceptual meaning. Criteria are designed with reference to the purposes for which the concept is being used and should be useful to both identify the concept and differentiate it from other concepts.

criteria for nursing diagnoses Essential features for a specific diagnosis to be used in a given instance or situation encountered in nursing practice.

critical reflection Process that questions the function, purposes, and value of empiric knowledge structures, especially theory, as reflected in the clarity, generality, simplicity, accessibility, and importance of the structure. The questioning process does not imply an expected response; for example, inquiring about clarity does not imply that clarity is desirable.

criticism A form of knowledge within the aesthetics pattern that is a discursive representation of meaning for expressions of aesthetic knowledge. Criticism is formed from aesthetic methods that are designed to deepen shared meanings for aesthetic knowing.

deduction Form of reasoning that moves from the general to the specific. In *deductive logic* two or more premises as relational statements are used to draw a conclusion; in *deductive research processes* an abstract theoretic relationship is used to derive specific questions or hypotheses.

definition Component of theory that indicates the empiric basis for a concept. Definitions are statements of meaning that provide a link between theoretic abstractions and empiric indicators. Definitions may be relatively general or specific.

deliberative application and validation of theory Theory development process that refines and develops empiric knowledge in relation to practice. Involves processes that refine conceptual meaning and validate theoretic relationships and outcomes within practice contexts.

descriptive relationships Statements that provide an account of what something is. Descriptive relationships provide an image or impression of the nature or attributes of a phenomenon.

dialogue Process of exchanging various points of view concerning what is right, good, or responsible. Interacts with the process of justification to challenge and authenticate ethical knowledge.

discipline Group of individuals engaged in developing a body of knowledge; the structured knowledge within an area of concern or domain of inquiry.

empiric-abstract continuum Means to visualize or represent the extent to which concepts have a basis in empiric reality. Empiric concepts have a direct reality basis and are more directly experienced, whereas abstract concepts have an indirect basis in empiric reality and are more mentally constructed.

empiric indicators The sensory experience related to a concept. More empirically grounded concepts have more direct empiric indicators; abstract concepts require the construction of indirect measures or tools that provide an approximate empiric measurement of some feature of the phenomenon.

empirics Fundamental pattern of knowing in nursing focused on the use of sensory experience for creation of mediated knowledge expressions. Expressed as knowledge by theories and models and integrated in practice as scientific competence.

envisioning Process of imagining forms, ways of being, actions, and outcomes into a possible future. Interacts with the process of rehearsing to create aesthetic knowledge.

epistemology Pertaining to the "stem" or basis of knowledge; perspectives on how knowing becomes knowledge or how knowledge is created.

ethics Fundamental pattern of knowing in nursing, focusing on matters of moral and ethical significance. Expressed as knowledge by principles and codes and integrated in practice as moral-ethical comportment.

explaining Process that focuses on how concepts and variables interrelate. Interacts with the process of structuring to create empiric knowledge.

explanatory relationships Statements that provide ideas about how events happen, indicating how related factors affect or result in certain phenomena.

fact Objectively verifiable event, object, or property; a phenomenon that is experienced and named similarly by others in a similar context.

general definition A statement of the meaning of a term or concept that sets forth characteristics of the phenomenon or what the phenomenon is associated with. A specific definition, by contrast, states particular characteristics, or indicators, that name what the phenomenon is.

generality Trait of theory useful for questioning, clarifying, and understanding the range of phenomena to which the theory applies. Generality combined with simplicity yields parsimony.

generalizability Extent to which research findings can be applied to or used as a basis for making decisions in like situations. Generalizability is affected by the soundness of the conceptualization process, the research design, and the analysis of the data.

genuine self A form of nondiscursive knowledge expression within the personal knowing pattern. Refers to the self, whole and entire, as understood by self and others.

grand theory Theory that deals with broad goals and concepts representing the total range of phenomena of concern within a discipline. This term may be used to imply macrotheory and molar and wholistic theory.

grounded theory Theory generated from inductive research processes; the source of data is empiric reality.

holism (see *wholism*)

holistic theory (see *wholistic theory*)

hypothesis Tentative statement of relationship between two or more variables that can be empirically tested. The term *hypothesis* is generally used to refer to a relationship statement that is tested by using specific research methods.

importance Trait of theory useful for questioning, clarifying, and understanding the extent to which a theory is clinically significant or has value for the profession.

induction Form of reasoning that moves from the specific to the general. In *inductive logic* a series of particulars are combined into a larger whole or set of things. In *inductive research* particular events are observed and analyzed as a basis for formulating general theoretic statements, often called *grounded theory.*

inspiration Process of responding to aesthetic knowledge to imagine new possibilities and directions. Interacts with appreciation to challenge and authenticate aesthetic knowledge.

isolated research Research that is completed without recognized reference or linkage to theory.

justification Process of developing explicit descriptions of the values on which an ethical ideal rests and the line of reasoning toward which an ethical conclusion flows. Interacts with the process of dialogue to challenge and authenticate ethical knowledge.

knowing Individual human processes of perceiving and understanding self and the world in ways that can be brought to some level of conscious awareness. Not all that is comprehended in the processes of knowing can be shared or communicated. What is shared, communicated, and expressed in words or in actions becomes the knowledge of a discipline.

knowledge Awareness or perception of reality acquired through insight, learning, or investigation expressed in a form that can be shared. Knowledge is a reasonably accurate accounting of the world as known and shared by members of a discipline. Knowledge is a representation of knowing that is collectively judged by shared standards and criteria.

law Relationship between variables that has been thoroughly tested and confirmed. Laws are said to be highly generalizable and are relatively certain.

logic System of reasoning that deals with the form of relationships among propositions without specific regard to their content.

macrotheory Theory that deals with a broad scope of phenomena. This term may be used to imply grand, molar, and wholistic theory.

metatheory Theory about the nature of theory and the processes for its development.

microtheory Theory that is relatively narrow in scope or deals with a narrow range of phenomena. This term may be used to imply atomistic and molecular theory.

midrange theory Substantive theory that tends to cluster around a concept (usually clinical) of interest to nursing; theories of pain alleviation, fatigue, or uncertainty represent theory in the midrange.

model Symbolic representation of empiric experience in words, pictorial or graphic diagrams, mathematical notations, or physical material (like a *model* airplane). A form of knowledge within the empirics pattern.

molar theory Theory that deals with a broad scope of phenomena. This term may be used to imply grand and wholistic theory and macrotheory.

molecular theory Theory that is relatively narrow in scope or deals with a narrow range of phenomena. This term may be used to imply microtheory and atomistic theory.

moral-ethical comportment Expression of ethical knowledge and knowing in nursing practice, integrated with personal, aesthetic, and empiric knowledge and knowing.

morals, morality The expression of ethical precepts in behavior and actions. Ontologic expression of what is good and right.

nursing practice Experiences a nurse encounters in the process of caring for people. Experiences include those of the person receiving care, the nurse, others in the environment, and their interactions.

objectivity Assumption on which methods of science are based, in which truth is thought to exist apart from or outside the person who knows. Based on a dualistic view of the rational mind and "out there" reality as separate.

ontology Pertaining to ways of being in the world; perspectives on the existence and experience of being.

opening Process that involves the taking in of experience fully and with conscious awareness. Interacts with the process of centering to create personal knowledge.

operational definition Statement of meaning that indicates how a term or concept can be assessed empirically. Operational definitions are inferred from theoretic definitions. They specify as exactly as possible the empiric indicators used to observe, assess, or measure the concept empirically. The standards or criteria to be used in making observations.

paradigm A worldview or ideology. A paradigm implies standards or criteria for assigning value or worth to both the processes and the products of a discipline, as well as for the methods of knowledge development within a discipline.

parsimony Trait of theory that incorporates degrees of both simplicity and generality. A highly parsimonious theory is one that has a broad range or generality yet is stated in very simple terms.

patterns gone wild The distortion of understanding that occurs when one pattern of knowing is not critically examined and integrated with the whole of knowing. Overemphasis on one pattern without integration leads to uncritical acceptance, narrow interpretations, and partial utilization of knowledge.

personal knowing Fundamental pattern of knowing in nursing focused on the inner experience of becoming a whole, aware self. Expressed as knowledge through autobiographic stories and the genuine self and integrated in practice with other patterns as therapeutic use of self.

philosophy Form of disciplined inquiry for the purpose of discerning general traits of reality and principles of value.

praxis Value-grounded, thoughtful reflection and action that occur in synchrony; integrates ontology and epistemology. Praxis constitutes nursing as a human caring practice and occurs when scientific competence, therapeutic use of self, moral-ethical comportment, and transformative art-acts occur in synchrony.

predicting Process used for the creation of empiric knowledge. Prediction involves a focus on interrelating concepts and variables to create understanding of when and how phenomena and events will occur and recur. Used in conjunction with explaining.

predictive relationships Set of statements that interrelates variables so that a specified outcome can be expected when the theory is used.

premises Relationship statements that are used in deductive logic as a basis for forming a conclusion. In logic the form of the argument must be valid, regardless of how sound the premises are. Examples of types of premises are hypotheses and axioms.

principles A form of knowledge expression within the ethics pattern. Principles are general statements that reflect general and fundamental precepts of value or truths that are followed in providing nursing care, such as "do no harm."

processes for theory development In a practice discipline the processes for theory development are creating conceptual meaning, structuring and contextualizing theory, refining and validating concepts and theoretic relationships, and deliberatively applying and validating theory.

profession Vocation that requires specialized knowledge, provides a role in society that is valued, and uses some means of internal regulations of its members.

proposition Statement of relationship between two or more variables. The term *proposition* is a general category that includes *postulates, premises, suppositions, axioms, conclusions, theorems,* and *hypotheses.* When a distinction in meaning is made between these various terms, the distinction reflects the form or purpose of logic used or the context in which the proposition occurs. For example, *hypothesis* is generally used in the context of a research study. *Axiom* and *theorem* are used to refer to the relationship statements that are made in a particular type of deductive logic.

purpose A component of theory that establishes reasons underlying a theory's development; the outcome or outcomes expected to emerge if the relationships of the theory are valid. The purpose of the theory also suggests the range of situations in which the theory is expected to apply.

reductionism Philosophic stance that the whole can be partitioned and understood through generalizations made from a study of the parts.

refining concepts and theoretical relationships A process for linking research and theory that focuses on the correspondence between the ideas of the theory and accessible experience that involves both qualitative and quantitative approaches. Includes validating empiric indicators for concepts, grounding emerging relationships empirically, and validating relationships through empiric methods.

reflection Process that requires integrating a wide range of perceptions in order to realize what is known within the self. Interacts with the process of response to challenge and authenticate personal knowledge.

rehearsing Process of creating and re-creating narrative, body movements, gestures, and actions in relation to an anticipated situation. Interacts with the process of envisioning to create aesthetic knowledge.

relationships Component of theory that refers to the interconnections between concepts.

relationship statements Any statement that sets forth a connection or association between two or more phenomena. This general term is used to denote both tentative and confirmed types of statements, such as propositions, laws, axioms, and hypotheses. As a more general term, it does not imply a particular form of logic or a particular context in which the statement is used.

replication Process that draws on methods of science to determine the extent to which an observation remains consistent from one situation or time to another. Interacts with the process of validation to challenge and authenticate empiric knowledge.

research Application of formalized methods of obtaining reliable and valid knowledge about empiric experience.

response Process of interacting with one's own self and others to provide insight concerning the meanings conveyed in experience. Interacts with the process of reflection to challenge and authenticate personal knowledge.

science As a product, the knowledge forms generated by the use of rigorous and precise empirically based methods, for example, facts, models and theories. As a process, the utilization of empirically based methods to generate theories, models, and descriptions of reality.

scientific competence Expression of empiric knowledge and knowing in nursing practice, integrated with ethics, aesthetics, and personal knowing and knowledge.

simplicity Trait of theory used in critical reflection for questioning, clarifying, and understanding the degree to which a theory reduces complexity by using a minimum number of descriptive components, especially concepts, to accomplish its purpose. Simplicity combined with generality yields parsimony.

specific definition Statement of the meaning of a term or concept that names the associated object, property, or event and assigns it particular characteristics, as opposed to saying what the concept is like or associated with in reality.

stories Tangible expression of personal knowledge that is discursive in form and that can be shared within the discipline.

structure A component of theory that refers to the overall morphologic arrangement of specific elements, especially concepts, within the theory.

structuring Process that involves forming empiric concepts into formal expressions such as theories, models, or frameworks. Interacts with the process of explaining to create empiric knowledge.

structuring and contextualizing theory Theory development process of forming relationships between and among concepts in a unique, creative, rigorous, and systematic way, consistent with the purposes of the theory. This process also includes identifying and defining the concepts, identifying assumptions, clarifying the context of the theory, and designing relationship statements.

theoretic definition Statement of meaning that conveys essential features of a concept in a manner that fits meaningfully within the theory. A theoretic definition specifies conceptual meaning and implies empiric indicators for concepts. This term may be used synonymously with *conceptual definition*.

theoretic framework A logical grouping of related concepts or theories, usually created to draw several different aspects together that are relevant to a complex situation such as a practice setting or an educational program. Term used synonymously with *conceptual framework*. A knowledge form within the empirics pattern.

theory An expression of knowledge within the empirics pattern. Creative and rigorous structuring of ideas that project a tentative, purposeful, and systematic view of phenomena.

theory-linked research Research that is designed with reference or linkage to theory. Theory-linked research may be theory testing or theory generating. *Theory-testing research* ascertains how accurately existing theoretic relationships depict reality-based events. *Theory-generating research* is designed to discover and describe relationships by observing empiric reality and then constructing theory based on empiric data observed.

therapeutic use of self Expression of personal knowledge and knowing in nursing practice, integrated with ethics and empiric and aesthetic knowledge and knowing.

transformative art-act Expression of aesthetic knowledge and knowing in nursing practice, integrated with empiric, aesthetic, and personal knowing and knowledge.

validation Process that draws on the methods of science to substantiate the accuracy of conceptual meanings in terms of empiric evidence. Interacts with replication to challenge and authenticate empiric knowledge.

values analysis A technique for objectively examining and seeking to understand the values operative in a situation as a basis for questioning the responsibleness of moral-ethical decisions.

values clarification A technique for subjectively examining, understanding, challenging, and embracing one's personal values. Values clarification provides a basis for questioning the responsibleness of moral-ethical decisions.

valuing Process of examining motives, actions, outcomes, and other dimensions of experience to embrace and reflect chosen values as a basis for understanding moral-ethical behavior. Interacts with the process of clarifying to create ethical knowledge.

wholism Perspective that is based on the assumption that a whole is emergent and cannot be reduced to discrete elements or be analyzed without residue into the sum of its parts. *Wholism* may also refer to an emphasis on the value of the whole but with consideration of discrete parts that are interrelated.

wholistic theory Theory that deals with a broad scope of phenomena. Use of the term *wholistic theory* often implies, in addition, an assumption that the whole is greater than the sum of its parts. This term may be used to imply macro and grand theory.

works of art Tangible expression of knowledge within the aesthetic patterns that is not discursive in form and that can be communicated and shared within the discipline. The term includes aesthetic expressions such as poetry, drawings, music, dance, and other forms of art as generally understood.

Index

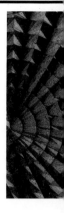